Herbal Medicine for Modern Life

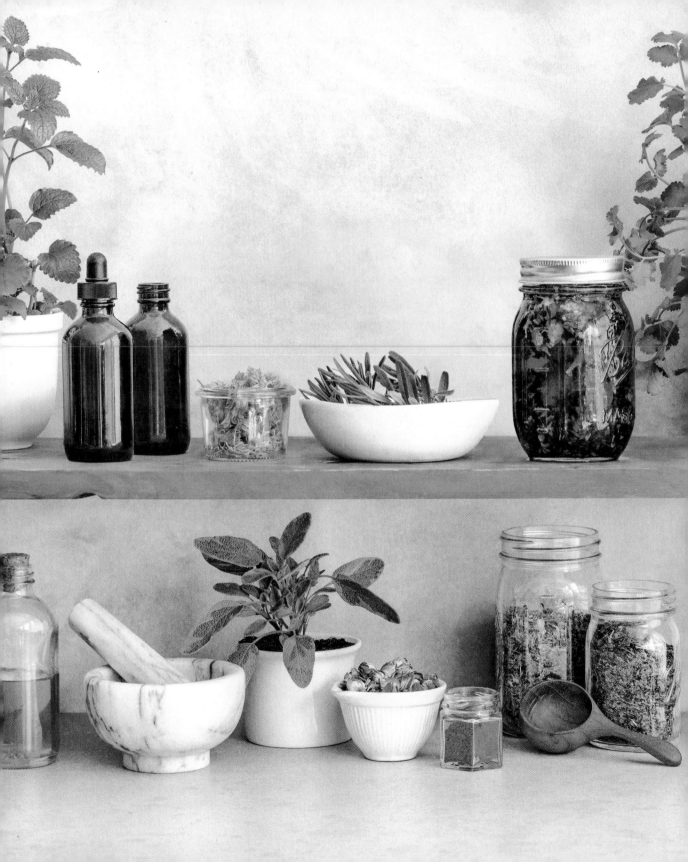

Herbal Medicine
for MODERN LIFE

Traditional Folk Remedies
for Everyday Health and Well-Being

Ruth A. Blanding

Photographs by Clare Barboza

ZEITGEIST • NEW YORK

The material in this book is for informational purposes only. It is not intended
to serve as a diagnostic tool or prescription manual, or to replace the advice
and care of your medical doctor. Although every effort has been made to
provide the most up-to-date information, medical science is rapidly changing.
Therefore, we strongly recommend that you consult your doctor before
attempting any of the treatments or programs discussed in this book. The
authors and publisher expressly disclaim responsibility for any adverse effects
that may result from the use or application of the information contained in
this book.

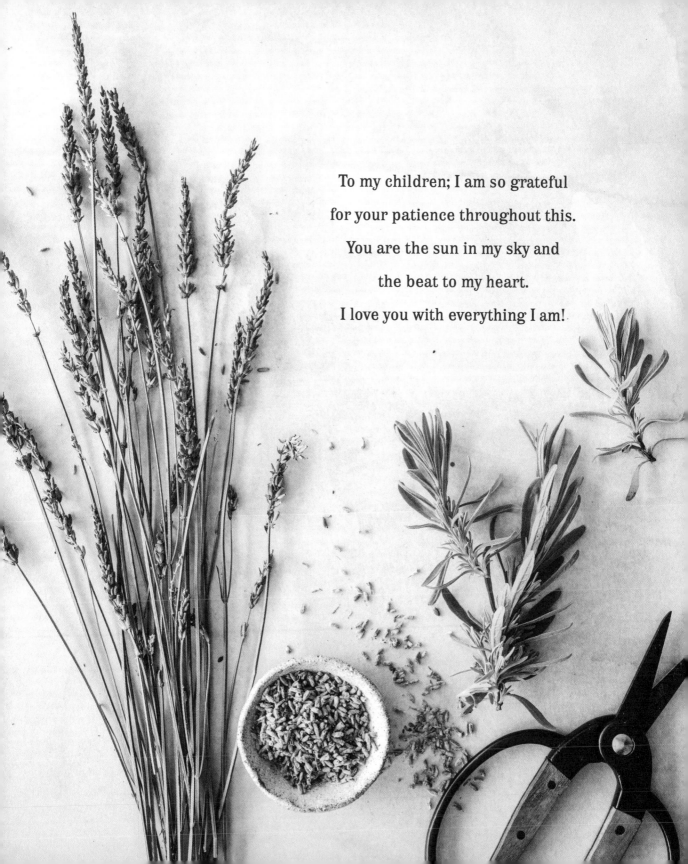

To my children; I am so grateful
for your patience throughout this.
You are the sun in my sky and
the beat to my heart.
I love you with everything I am!

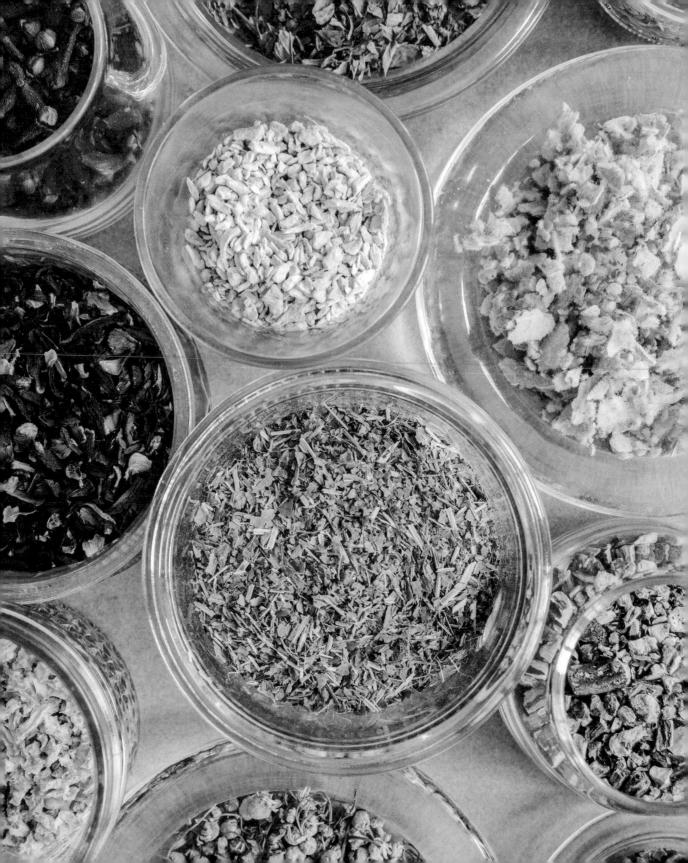

Contents

Part III
HERBAL FOLK REMEDIES FOR MODERN AILMENTS

COMFREY

Protecting against Environmental and Lifestyle Stressors

Addressing Pharmaceutical and Dietary Effects

Managing Physical Pain and Discomfort

Managing Respiratory Illnesses and Allergies

Supporting Sexual and Reproductive Health

Treating Digestive Issues

Support for Chronic Conditions

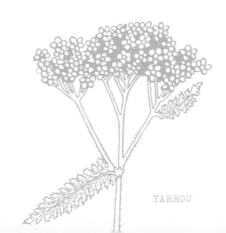

YARROW

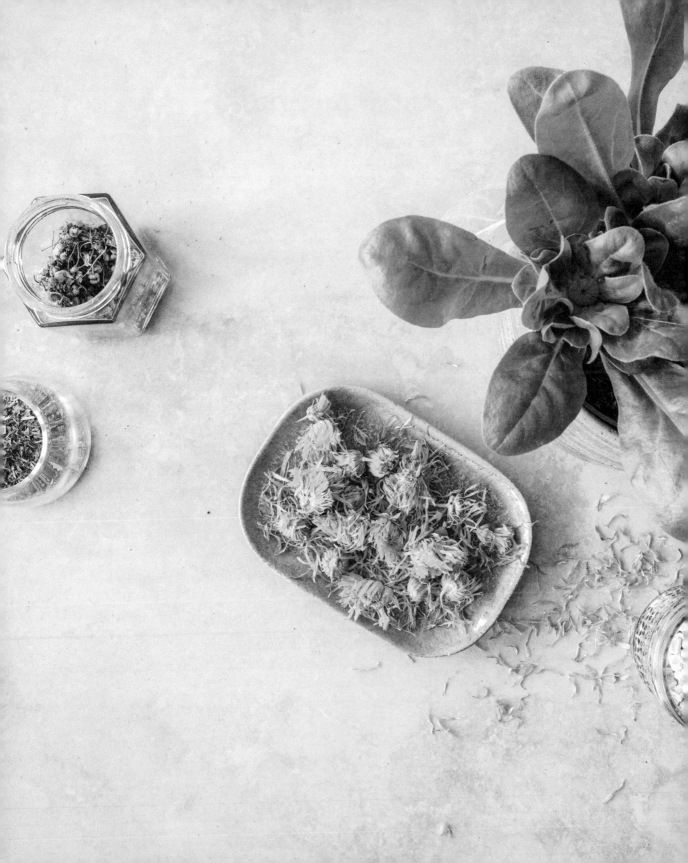

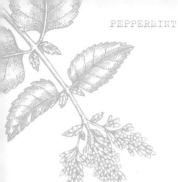

Introduction

Hello, dear friends. I am so excited to welcome you to the wonderful world of herbal folk remedies. As we journey through these pages, I am here to be both your guide and your fellow explorer. Whether you have been dabbling in herbal medicine for a while or are new to these practices, let us all meet as equals.

I began my herbal journey more than twenty years ago as a teenager seeking knowledge outside the four walls of Western allopathic medicine. To deepen my connection to the Earth and her Sacred gifts, I began to listen and speak to plants, whom I view as respected teachers. Like my ancestors before me, I have worked hard to understand their language and learn their powerful lessons. I care as much for the plants who nourish us in our day-to-day lives as the Sacred medicines who heal us in ceremonies. I have meandered through the garden of knowledge that is herbalism and, even after all these years, I remain a humble and joyful student of herbal traditions and medicine.

This book is a beginner-friendly guide to practicing and crafting your own herbal home remedies. Within these pages, I will share a collection of herbal traditions, practices, and remedies that can be used in your everyday life. From simple teas to tinctures and salves, we will unwrap the gifts that our herbal allies have to share. Along the way, you may gain a deeper connection to and understanding of the herbs themselves and what they want to teach you, all while becoming less reliant on the use of conventional Western medicines.

As we embark on this journey together, I want to ask you to take a moment to honor the power of herbs and herbal medicines. Medicinal herbs are generally quite safe, but not every herb is safe for every person. We are all graced with a unique inner universe, and herbal medicine will have a different effect on each of us because of this. This means it is always wise to speak with professionals when beginning your herbal remedies and medicinals journey. And for those who are using conventional allopathic medications, consult your physician before using any herbs to make sure you are not mixing herbal and allopathic medicine in a way that could place your health and well-being in danger.

Together, we will explore dozens of herbal folk remedy recipes that will address a multitude of common symptoms, ailments, discomforts, and conditions that many people seek relief for. We will discover the hidden treasures and ancient wisdom of many plant and herbal allies to support ease and health in our modern lives.

Thank you, dear friend, for joining me on this journey. May the sun ever shine on your garden and may the rain bring about bountiful medicine.

Your friend,
Ruth A. Blanding

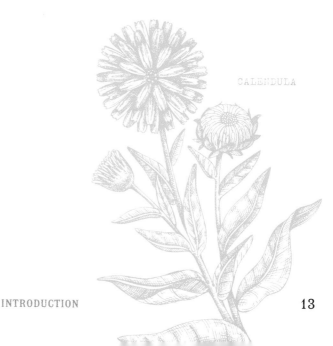

CALENDULA

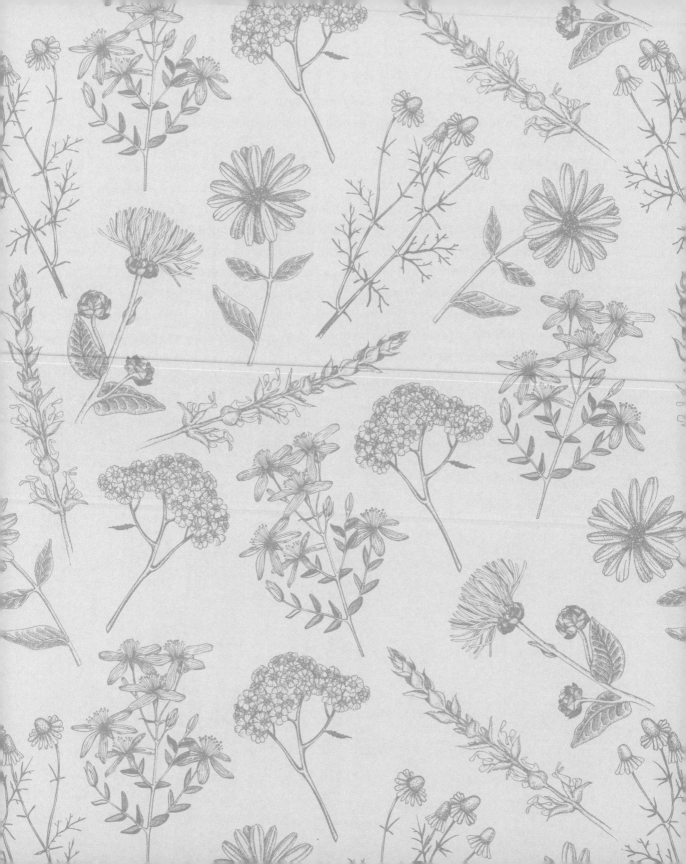

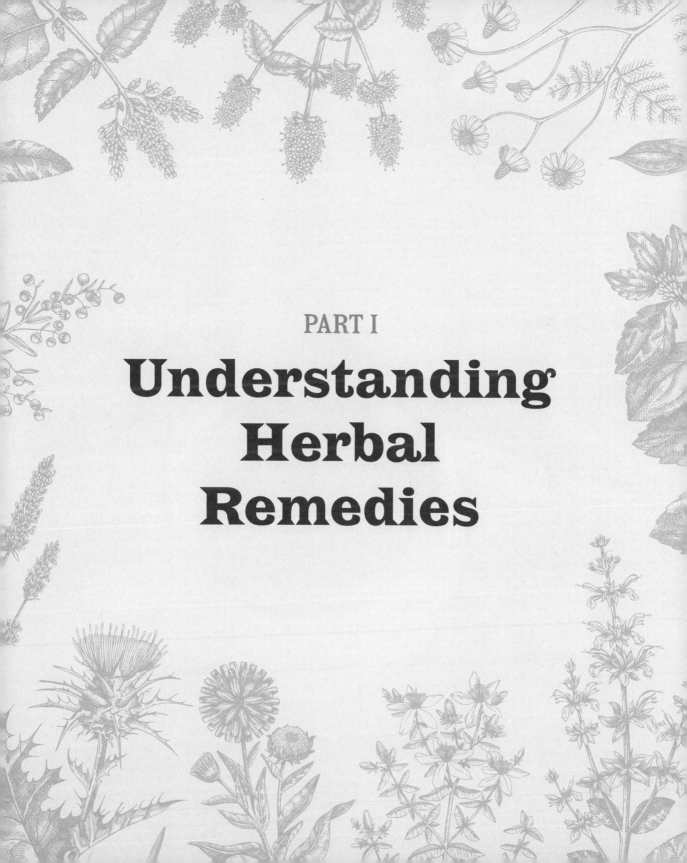

PART I

Understanding Herbal Remedies

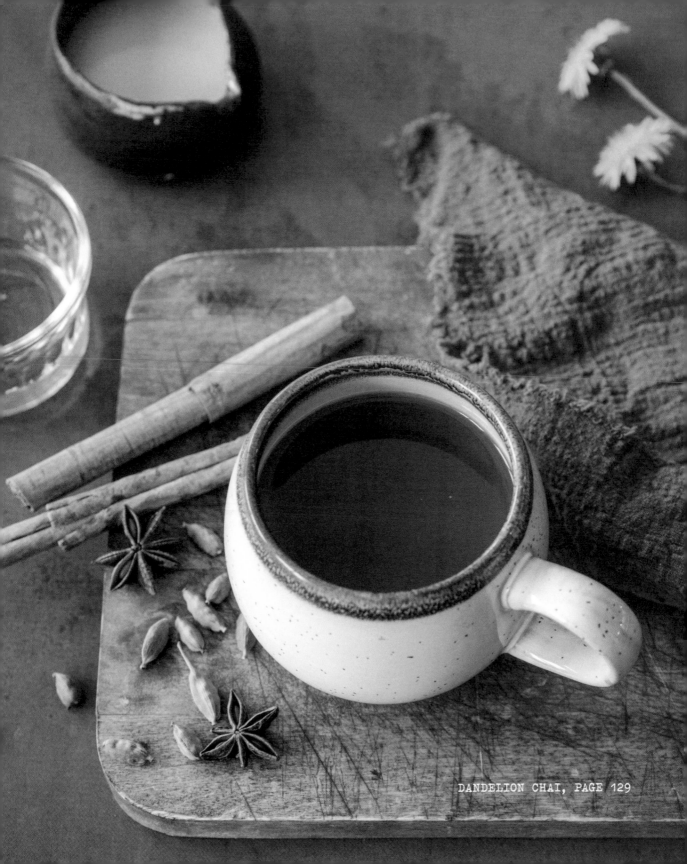

DANDELION CHAI, PAGE 129

1

FROM FOLK MEDICINE
TO HERBAL MEDICINE

To me, folk remedies and herbalism are the anchor points of our healing practices. They are the lifeblood of humanity, reaching from the past into the future. They are beautiful and ancient living arts. They are healing crafts passed down from generation to generation. They are ever-evolving and yet never change; there is a deep and abiding comfort in that. Folk remedies and herbalism are the backbone upon which our Western allopathic medicinal practices are built. And, to me, they are the key to whole wellness.

Folk Medicine and Traditional Medicine

You might be asking yourself what folk medicine is and what it has to do with herbalism and your modern health needs. Folk medicine is structured around Indigenous traditional physiology and healing wellness practices that have been passed down from person to person, usually within a family or tight-knit community. Much of the knowledge is specific to individual cultural traditions, locations/regions, and practices. It is passed down orally and through hands-on learning in apprentice-style relationships—grandmother to granddaughter, elder to youth.

Folk medicine is practiced all around the world. Some forms you might be familiar with are African root work, Arabic Unani/Yunani, Ayurveda, traditional Chinese medicine, and the Sacred practices of the Indigenous American people. These practices are deeply steeped in the spiritual and the energetic, as much as they are in the physical and the physiological. As an Afro-Indigenous person, I have drawn on and combined the knowledge of my heritage to create a blend of African and Indigenous American folk remedies that will, one day, be passed down to my own children as a new branch of folk medicine.

Every single one of us has folk medicine in our heritage. If you did not grow up with the experience of having healing knowledge shared with you, you can become the creator of that knowledge for the next generation of your family. In developing your library of remedies, you will become the bridge from the past to the future!

Challenges and Obstacles to Practicing Herbal Medicine

In our busy modern-day lifestyle, it can be increasingly difficult to practice folk and traditional medicine because, often, it is so much easier to just grab ready-made medications. We are a generation of people who have become quite time-poor, moving from one task to the other with very little room to think about anything in between. Caring for our minds and bodies often takes the hit. Many people feel as though traditional remedies are inaccessible, and that too many obstacles stand between themselves and having an easeful relationship with these practices.

Some obstacles that people have mentioned to me personally include:

* Lack of reputable information online
* High cost of premade remedies
* Uncertainties about who to ask for help, aside from their allopathic doctors
* Concern about harmful interactions with their prescribed medications
* Lack of energy to learn a new skill

I know starting a new health journey can feel like an uphill battle, but I want to take a moment to ease your mind. Although the just-noted obstacles are valid, there are *absolutely* ways for everyone to practice herbal medicine, including those people struggling to know just where and how to begin. In this book, I walk with you hand in hand as you learn how to add this practice to your daily life. And by the final page, it is my hope that you will have a nourishing and joy-filled relationship with plant medicine.

Herbalism and Herbal Medicine

Herbalism. You have probably heard the term a million times but may still wonder exactly what it is and why it might be important to your health and wellness. The short answer is that herbalism is the practice of working with plants as medicine for ailments of all kinds. It has been practiced for as long as humans have been sentient beings. It is such a common part of human culture that most people don't even realize they practice it in one form or another every day. Do you take a cup of chamomile tea for stress, or peppermint when you are stuffy? Congratulations! You, my friend, are practicing herbalism.

Herbal medicine is the more structured and systemized way to interact with herbs. Have you gone to the market and purchased an herbal salve for cuts or arnica rub for bruises? Have you used chaste tree tinctures to stimulate ovulation or taken a holistic cough syrup for a chest cold? Now you are practicing herbal medicine. At the end of the day, they are two sides of the same coin: working with plant allies to assist in soothing the discomforts and illnesses we all face and also increasing our pleasurable, self-care moments. There are no barriers or restrictions when it comes to who practices herbal medicine—it is as much the domain of the urban youth and the high-stakes business professional as it is the country grandmother. Herbal medicine is a global connecting point that spans cultures, classes, and abilities. Though each culture has Sacred, special, and unique ways in which they honor, respect, commune with, and work with herbal allies, this practice is something all of our ancestors have in common.

So what is the relationship between herbalism and folk medicine? Folk medicine is not limited to working with herbs and plant allies. It incorporates a vast array of energetic interactions (such as connecting to chi energy), spiritual connection (such as speaking to our ancestors for guidance), and working with natural substances to accelerate healing (such as spreading clay on the skin to remove impurities or putting onions on the feet to pull congestion from the chest). Each collection of folk medicine remedies is as diverse as the people who practice them and the places they are practiced. What they all have in common, though, is that, in some capacity, all folk medicine practices incorporate herbalism into their healing processes.

An Increasingly Popular Approach

While herbalism and the practice of herbal medicine have, in one capacity or another, been part of the human experience since before recorded history, recent years have witnessed a major boom in the adoption of herbalism and herbal medicine in both personal and professional contexts. Some people may be curious as to why these practices have suddenly increased in popularity in our modern society. I have two main theories:

1. On one hand, people are sick and tired of feeling sick and tired. Many allopathic medications have a laundry list of side effects, ranging from mild discomfort to secondary negative health conditions. No one wants to feel sick while trying to feel better.

2. Another possibility is that there has been a massive increase in the number of chronic illnesses that people are suffering from. More and more, people are being diagnosed with allergies, asthma, eczema, gut disorders, and other ongoing conditions. Many of these are caused by exposure to harmful chemicals in our environment, our food, and our water sources. I believe that people are looking back to find their way forward.

Our ancestors survived and thrived while working with ingredients and remedies that came from the Earth. There are records of plants and herbs helping to stave off pregnancy as well as easing tooth pain and supporting oral health. Not only were our ancestors working with plant allies as a regular part of their existence, but cultures across the world relied on plants with similar qualities for similar purposes. For instance, peppermint is grown natively in Eurasia, North America, Southern Africa, and Australia and people in all of these places work with it to ease nausea and gastrointestinal upset. Herbalism and herbal medicine really make the world go round!

"Magic, Spirit, and Energy"

As we delve into the wonders and the details of folk and traditional medicine practices, I want to take a moment to touch on the deep connection among plant medicine, energy work, and Earth magic belief systems. Folk and traditional medicinal practices are not simply about healing the body—they are about full systemic health. They are also about building intimate connections to the plants and natural materials that are our partners in this work. For many who practice folk and traditional medicine, both today and in the time of our ancestors, each plant (in truth, every aspect of the natural world) possesses energetic life and sentience. Plants are spoken to and treated as wise and honored relatives. Often while learning the path of plant medicine, students are encouraged to sit and listen to the plants, to hear what they want to teach us and learn in what ways the plants want to be "in relationship" with us as individual practitioners. In this way, the new practitioner learns to be present with our plant family. It is to this energy that spiritual beliefs and the concepts of magic are tied.

Within specific cultural and ethnic communities of folk and traditional medicine practices, there are plants designated as Sacred. Though I know it is not always possible, it is the goal that Sacred plants be used only within these groups and for specific ceremonies, prayers, rituals, and medicine creation. In many Indigenous American communities, the four Sacred plants are cedar, sage, sweetgrass, and tobacco. In African Diasporic plant medicine practices, boneset, cotton root, and mullein are highly revered. In Ayurvedic practices, plants of spiritual significance are ashoka, bilva, peepal, sandalwood, and tulsi.

MULLEIN

Appreciating these cultural nuances may be new to you and feel confusing or awkward at first. Nevertheless, I ask that you strive to respect the beliefs, practices, and traditions of plant medicine and its practitioners as well as honor the Sacred plants, and find alternatives to work with during your folk medicine journey.

Though we do not need science to validate what is known to be truth within the folk and traditional medicine communities, sometimes it is fun to note when science "catches up" to the old ways. In recent years, science has proven what so many throughout time have always known: that plants can speak and hear in their own way. They can engage, and they can affect their environments as much as they can be affected by events in their environments.

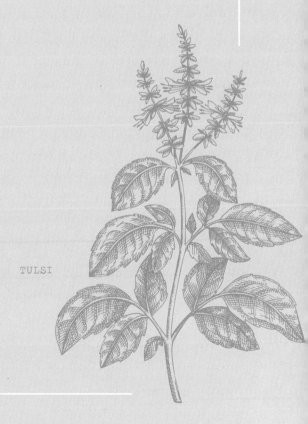

TULSI

Why Try Herbal Folk Remedies?

There are a million and one reasons I would recommend trying herbal folk remedies, especially in today's high-stress, low-rest society. Since I can't possibly fit them all into this book, here are some of the top reasons I believe herbal folk remedies should become part of your life!

1. *They are simple.* An herbal remedy is as simple or as complex as the crafter wants it to be. Many single-herb remedies can be used to treat a wide array of ailments. For example, nettles—as a tea, a tincture, or a supplement—can treat allergies, arthritis (including gout), and inflammation and help calibrate an overtaxed nervous system.

2. *They are cost-effective.* For the most part, herbs are sold by weight, and (outside of some hard-to-access or hard-to-grow herbs such as vanilla) are fairly inexpensive. If you have a small amount of space and the ability to grow herbs in a pot or planter or on a windowsill, you can access your plant medicine at virtually no cost.

3. *They can be shared.* Unlike allopathic medication, plant medicine is meant to be shared. In many of the places I have lived, it has been common practice for local herbalists to craft large quantities of fire ciders, elderberry syrups, smoke-ease teas (for fire-prone areas), and immune support blends (especially since the start of the COVID-19 pandemic) and offer them to the community for free or for a minimal fee.

4. *They are multipurpose.* One herb can have many talents. Turmeric is an herb that can seem almost mythical in its healing properties, treating allergies, arthritis, depression, digestive disorders, liver disease, respiratory infections, and so much more.

5. *You know the source and the ingredients.* When you are crafting your own herbal remedies, you *always* know the source of your medicine and what ingredients are in your remedies. This is not always the case with store-bought or prescription medicines.

6. *They offer autonomy.* When you begin your folk remedy journey, you actively take control of your health and wellness in a way that is often challenging when dealing with allopathic medicine and doctors in the healthcare system.

7. *They create empowerment of self.* As a practitioner of herbal remedies, you decide how your health story is going to unfold.

8. *They are accessible.* Not everyone has access to medical insurance, but nearly everyone has access to herbs through grocery stores, farmer's markets, or your own backyard.

9. *They offer complementary/collaborative care to allopathic medicine.* Choosing to work with plant medicine and folk remedies does not mean avoiding allopathic medicinal care. You can improve your knowledge and your health by working alongside your doctor to make sure you do not take herbs that will react negatively with your allopathic medications.

Ancient Remedies for Modern Life

In my work as a traditional herbalist, plant medicine practitioner, and life-long student of plant medicine, I find that I am taking a journey toward my ancestors, and thus more fully and deeply into myself. Though I speak about remedies and practices from many different cultures, I lean most heavily on the traditions of my Indigenous American and African American heritages. These remedies are intertwined with some of the original stories of the land upon which we all live in North America; they are the first conversations between my people and our plant relatives, and to be able to learn this tongue, to be able to join this conversation, makes me feel like I am a time traveler. It also makes me feel a satisfying connection to my roots and the knowledge that has always been mine, waiting for me to rediscover it.

About the Remedies

When selecting remedies would for this book, I had a few simple criteria. First and foremost, these remedies needed to address conditions associated with modern living—things such as environmental health disruption, chronic health conditions, and maladies of high-stress, low-rest living. Secondly, I wanted the remedies to be simple enough that anyone could craft them with minimal time and effort. Many of us today have a limited time in our day for new activities, and I wanted to make it as easy as possible for anyone to begin and maintain a plant medicine and folk remedies practice. Thirdly, and probably most important to me, these recipes needed to be simultaneously accessible and culturally respectful. Too often in the world of natural health and wellness, it can feel as though information is tailored to people who look a certain way, or believe certain things, or who have lots of money and time. I wanted to make it clear that plant medicine is for everyone, so I chose remedies that can be created and used by everyone. Finally, I wanted the remedies I share to encourage every person who picks up this book to get curious and explore writings and folk remedy knowledge from their personal ancestry. It is by honoring the knowledge of our ancestors and our heritage that we learn to honor and respect the knowledge of others. And in honoring our history, we understand not to blindly take from cultures that are not ours.

I also chose remedies that I knew to be effective. For the most part, and for most people, plant medicine and folk remedies are incredibly safe and effective. Most of the ingredients in this book's recipes are crafted with plants and herbs that are already in many people's kitchen pantries. As with anything that you put on or in your body, it is important to understand what the possible harmful side effects are. I suggest that you research potential side effects and allergy information for the herbs you intend to work with. It is also important to know what your sensitivities are. For instance, are you allergic to ragweed or daisies? If so, chamomile might trigger an allergic reaction. This is because all three of these flowers are part of the Asteraceae family and so can trigger similar allergic reactions. The more aware you are, the safer you are. And if you take allopathic medications or over-the-counter drugs, *always* check to make sure the herb you take will not adversely react to the medications in your system. When in doubt, ask an herbal and/or medical professional.

As to the question of efficacy, this will depend on the herb/herbs and the constitution of the person working with them. Some people may be incredibly sensitive to the effects of a certain remedy and feel a shift immediately, whereas others may have a higher threshold and take longer to feel the effects. With herbal medicines and folk remedies, depending on the herbs and how they are being worked with, effects may become noticeable anywhere from three days to three months later. Not every remedy will work for every person. If you do not feel as though a certain remedy is working for you, that is okay! Get curious! What are similar remedies or herbal allies with similar effects that could work? Herbal medicine and folk remedies are all about experimentation and learning the delicate dance, the conversation, between yourself and the plant medicine.

About the Ailments

In planning which ailments to address in this book, I wanted to touch on whole systems as well as the specific illnesses and life stressors that affect those systems. So, throughout the book, I follow this approach:

1. We will talk about how to engage with herbal medicine and folk remedies to protect against environmental stressors such as poor air quality, smoke inhalation from wildfires, and unremediated household mold.

2. We will explore using herbal medicines and folk remedies to mitigate the side effects of pharmaceutical treatments. This includes ways to boost gut biome, reduce nausea, and increase appetite when allopathic medications have disrupted comfortable function.

3. We will discuss managing physical pain and discomfort brought on by both intermittent illness and chronic disorders.

4. We will talk about remedies for allergies and respiratory illnesses including COVID, asthma, and general upper-respiratory congestion.

5. We will hold respectful space as we discuss how to support the reproductive health system for *all* people. Among the topics we will touch on will be how to support menstrual disorders, hormone replacement therapy (HRT) discomfort, infertility, and decreased or diminishing sex drive.

6. We will be gentle in our conversation around caring for ourselves, including our mental and emotional health needs. We will discuss finding ways to ease the symptoms, if not the presence, of anxiety, depression, and insomnia as well as safe ways to support any allopathic medications that help mitigate these disorders.

7. We will learn which herbs can be helpful in supporting and treating digestive issues such as acid reflux/gastroesophageal reflux disease (GERD), celiac disease, Crohn's disease, irritable bowel syndrome (IBS), and leaky gut syndrome.

8. We will learn how to treat—and, in some instances, work to clear—bacterial and fungal overgrowths such as candida.

9. And we will find ways in which herbal medicine and folk remedies can support a more easeful life for people living with chronic conditions such as fibromyalgia, heart disease, and weak or compromised immune systems.

It is my goal for each remedy in this book to help facilitate health, to help ease discomfort, and to help you learn to care for your health through folk remedies and plant ally medicines.

What to Expect

As we move forward together in this herbal journey, I want to touch on expectations and realities around herbal and folk remedies. Plants and herbs can do amazing things. Yet while folk remedies and herbal medicine are powerful, these remedies are not meant as cure-alls. They are a guidepost, a starting point, and a support structure that that will assist you in your health and wellness journey.

I am excited to move with you further into this conversation around the bountiful offerings of our plant allies. In the next chapter, we will begin the work of building your confidence as an herbal medicine practitioner. I'll prepare you to go from a person in search of answers to a person crafting their own care with the aid of plant and folk remedies.

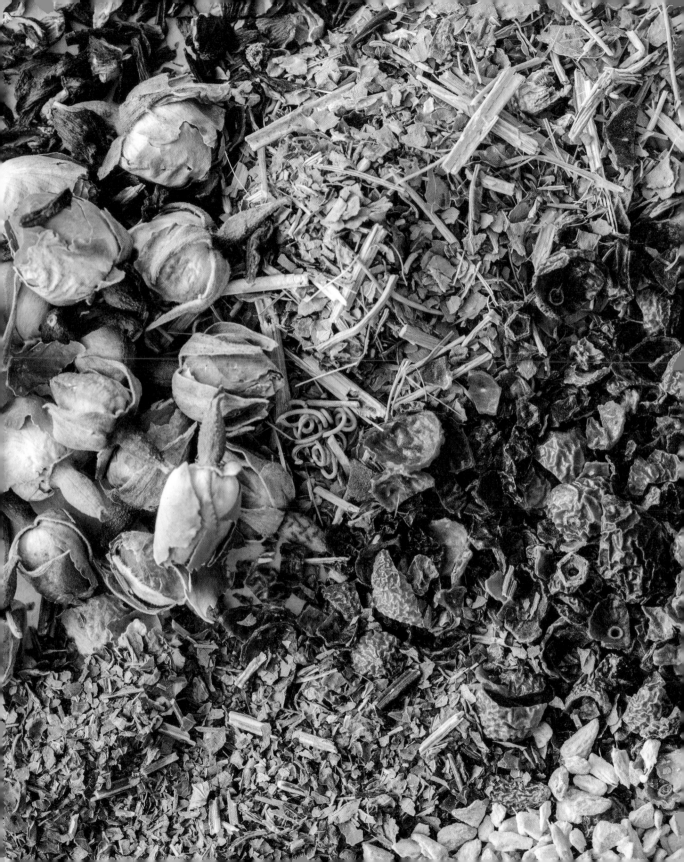

2

WORKING WITH
HERBAL MEDICINE

You've made it! Welcome to working with herbal medicine. All the joy of herb crafting begins with the steps you'll find in this chapter. Here, we are going to dive into where and how to source your herbs and the supplies you may need for crafting your folk remedies and herbal medicines. From understanding how to practice herb crafting safely to protecting at-risk plant allies to learning safe dosages and more, I walk with you on the path to becoming well-rounded in the art of herbal medicine creation.

Sourcing Medicinal Plants

Learning how and where to source your herbs can be a nerve-wracking experience. There are so many options—both online and in person—that it can be hard to know which way to go and whom to trust. Here are some of the steps I use to source the best herbs possible:

Aim for Local First There is nothing quite like walking into an herbal apothecary for the first time. The jars filled with greenery and colorful buds, the scent of herbs wafting through the air, the almost-palpable energy of endless possibilities. And the often super friendly and knowledgeable shopkeepers ready and waiting to assist you. Truly, if you have the luxury of access to a local shop, use it. There is nothing like meeting the herbs in person to get a feel for which ones you wish to work with. And the ability to ask questions, be in conversation, and build relationships with your local herb professionals is worth its weight in roses!

Check for Freshness This is such a key part of crafting folk remedies and herbal medicines. Fresh herbs make the most potent medicine! How do you know if something is fresh? If you have a local shop, ask. Most shopkeepers are happy to share this information with you. The next step is to use your senses to check out the herbs. Look: Does the herb have good color? Is it vibrant green or dull and faded? Are the flowers dried properly or do they feel damp or appear moldy? Smell: This works best for in-person buying but is also important for online orders that may need to be returned. Is there a strong herbal scent when you open the containers? If the scent is dull or difficult to detect, chances are the herbs are at the end of their usability. Taste: Ask the shopkeeper if you can take a small sample beforehand in case there is a specific way they want you to handle the herbs. Is there a strong flavor? It might be sweet, spicy, pungent, sharp, aromatic, salty, or bitter. A strong flavor is a good sign that the herbs are fresh.

Learn the Lingo of the Label When buying herbs, you may come across some vague terminology such as "fair trade," "natural," "organic," "sustainable," or "wildcrafted." Let me clarify what those terms mean so you can shop for herbs with confidence.

- When a supplier states their herbs are fair trade, it means the herbs are sourced through a certified company that has a relationship with farmers living in globally marginalized countries. It requires that growers not only receive a fair and just wage but also funding to put back into their communities or businesses.

- The label "natural" doesn't offer any real information. Sometimes companies will use this word as a way to say that the plant was grown in a clean, chemical-free way. However, for me, this is not enough information to really know how the herbs were grown or handled before they got to market.

- Organic herbs are grown using only organic materials, with no pesticides or chemicals, on unpolluted land. There are multiple certifying bodies, the most familiar being the USDA, that help guarantee that a company is following very specific practices to be classified and certified as organic.

- An herb labeled "sustainable" means that the practices used in growing, harvesting, transporting, and selling this herb not only preserve biological diversity but also help in the regeneration of the ecosystem in which the herb is grown. Not only is the growing of the herb important, but the treatment of the growers is of equal relevance. Sustainable growing practices support and enhance cultural diversity, economic equity in the form of fair livable wages, and respectful treatment for everyone involved, including our planet.

- Wildcrafted herbs are picked in their wild, natural habitat. This is also called foraging. Wildcrafted herbs, when grown in areas unharmed by pollutants, often are of a higher quality and potency than their farmed counterparts. It is important to know whether your wildcrafted herbs are foraged following sustainable guidelines since overforaging an area can cause habitat damage.

Know the Harvesting Practices I am a bit of a stickler when it comes to knowing where my herbs were sourced and what practices were used in their harvesting process. Why is the harvesting process so important? Because some herbs need to be harvested in specific ways to ensure they maintain their medicinal properties and potency. Harvesting at the right time of year, in the right phase of the plant's life cycle, in the right weather, along with knowing how the herbs are handled before and during the drying processes and the storing and packaging processes, all contribute to the quality of the herb.

Know the Storage Practices Another important aspect of the herb sourcing process is knowing how the herbs are stored. Herbs do best in cool, dark, airtight containers and environments. Keeping light exposure to a minimum helps keep the herbs fresh. Heat damages herbs, so it is best to keep the space where your herbs are stored under 100°F. If you are shopping for your herbs online, especially if you order loose-packaged or bulk, you will most likely receive your herbs in plastic bags. Feel free to contact the company and ask how the herbs are stored before they are placed in bags in preparation for shipping. Every business is different, so it is important to ask.

For Online Stores, Read the Reviews It is never easy to buy something online, and the process is even more complex than usual when it comes to herbs and plant medicine. My best practice suggestion is to find potential herb companies by first searching for your required standards of practice (such as BIPOC owned/operated, eco-sustainable, fair trade, locally sourced, organic, wildcrafted, etc.) and then doing a little digging. Read the company's sustainability practices statement, which should be on their website. Also read the reviews. If a business has unethical practices or poor-quality herbs, people will talk!

Make Herb Friends and Talk to the Local Herbal Medicine Community
If there is one thing I know for sure, it is that practicing herbal medicine and learning about folk remedies is most fulfilling when you have other enthusiasts around you. Jump into a local herb group! Join an online herb community! These are your people. They can help you find the best sources for herbs as well as the best deals.

Support Underrepresented Herb Suppliers I cannot emphasize this strongly enough: Sourcing herbs from growers from underrepresented communities not only adds diversity to your home herbal apothecary, but also increases the diversity of your herbal community. There are many herb suppliers from underrepresented communities such as AAPI/NHAOPI (Asian American, Pacific Islander, Native Hawaiian, Asian, Other Pacific Islander), BBIA (Black, Brown/Latinx, Indigenous, Asian), and LGBTQIA+ who are doing big work in growing unique heirloom herbs as well as herbs that are culturally and ethnically important.

Start with Small Batch Orders Another must for me in herb sourcing is knowing where and how to get a good price. The best way to do this is to order in small batches instead of bulk orders. Small batches are generally a few ounces and let you try an herb without committing to a huge amount. Once you know that you like an herb, that it works for you, and that you want to keep it on hand, grab some in bulk. But remember to buy only what you will need in the amount of time the herb will stay fresh.

Try your best to buy from reputable sources only, which may include a local herbalist or local herb shop, the local natural foods store, or online shops that have been vetted and reviewed. At the end of the day, it comes down to doing your digging. Asking people in your online community, reading online reviews, checking websites certifications, and reading about the herb farmers a seller works with all are ways to source herbs and plants safely for your remedies.

When shopping online, search around for the deals. Nearly every herb-supplying website I have used has a sale or deals page. Check there first! You might find exactly what you need, and even some things you didn't know you needed but can now afford, at really great prices. Also join their newsletter! This is where news about upcoming sales, flash sales, and discount coupons will be. I even have a separate address for these promotional emails so I don't miss the deals. Check out the resource page at the back of the book for websites for my favorite tried, true, and trusted herbal suppliers.

These nine steps comprise the foundation to making herb purchasing a stress-free experience, which gives me the freedom to happily craft my herbal medicine. Happy sourcing!

Common Preparations to Buy

Making your own folk remedies and herbal medicines is definitely the goal. But sometimes time and life get full and you may need to buy a quick remedy. Here are some remedies you can purchase online, access in store, or make easily at home.

Teas Teas are probably the simplest and most common way that herbal medicine is crafted. They can be made from a single herb or a complex combination of multiple herbs thoughtfully mixed for their combined healing properties. Teas can be made from fresh or dried herbs.

Capsules As the name suggests, this form of herbal medicine is contained in tiny cylindrical containers, which are usually made from a vegan or vegetarian material such as tapioca, and filled with finely processed herbs. Similar to teas, capsules can contain a single dried herb or multiple dried herbs thoughtfully mixed for their combined healing properties.

Tinctures and Extracts Tinctures are concentrated herbal extractions that have an alcohol base, whereas extracts are concentrated herbal extractions using other solvents such as water, vinegar, or glycerin. They can be made from single herbs or multiple herb blends.

Syrups and Elixirs Syrups are often made by cooking down the herbal or plant material and then adding honey as a sweetener. Elixirs are sweetened herbal liquids that are made using both alcohol and water. Both can be used to help ease discomfort and symptoms of illness as well as support health.

You can purchase herbal teas, tinctures, extracts, capsules, syrups, and elixirs online at suppliers such as Mountain Rose Herbs (one of my favorites), Frontier Co-Op, and Starwest Botanicals, and in person at local herb shops and even natural food stores such as Erewhon (Los Angeles County, California), Good Earth Market (Marin County, California), Sprouts Farmers Market, and Whole Foods Market (throughout the United States).

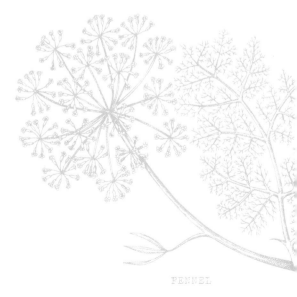

FENNEL

Protecting At-Risk Plants

As you move further toward becoming a conscientious steward of plant medicine, I want to speak to you about at-risk plants. Overforaging has become frustratingly common in the commercial herbal market. Every time an herb becomes the new "it" medicine, the market gets saturated with products relying on that herb as an ingredient. This causes major disruption to the growth and safety of that plant. And many times, overharvesting an herb can cause immense harm to the plants in its native growing environment as well as put the herb at risk of extinction. It is the responsibility of each and every one of us who works with plant medicine to protect the herbs and plant allies that help us craft our medicines. We can do this in many ways:

- Substitute other herbs that have the same or similar effects for the at-risk herb.
- Don't overforage if you have access to the plant in its native habitat.
- Gather only exactly as much as you need for personal/individual purposes.
- Source locally.
- Source only from sustainable and reputable suppliers, and check their standards, practices, and certifications.
- Grow what you can! I know that it's a privilege to have the space and time to grow your own medicine. But if you can, do it! You will have exactly what you want and need available, and you can begin to build a truly intimate relationship with your plant.

There are many groups that work diligently to protect native herbs and their habitats. You can find some of these groups listed in the resource section of this book.

ECHINACEA

Best Practices

If you are anything like me, any time you start something new, you go all out and buy *everything* you could possibly ever need for your new activity or practice. When it comes to my personal herbal practice, however, I work in the opposite direction. To get the most out of my practice, here are some simple steps I follow:

1. Start small! I can't stress this enough. Start with one or two herbs or simple recipes. What do you need right now for your health and wellness? It takes time to build a healthy and functional home apothecary. There is no need to rush. Grow your store of medicine slowly and with love!

2. Order herbs in small batches. Doing so means you will enjoy your herbs at their peak.

3. Craft only what you need. One of the best ways to craft remedies sustainably is to make only what you will use in the immediate future. This helps guarantee that your medicines are at their highest potency when you take them and, if we each do our part, has a positive impact on how plants are harvested and sold in the herbal market.

4. Set aside a cool, dark, dry space for your herbs. This could be a space in your kitchen cupboards, in your closet, or in a special hutch or shelf.

5. Read, learn, gather, grow! Get to know your herbs. Ask questions and get curious. Crafting herbal medicines and folk remedies is an art and a practice. Play and have fun and your skills will blossom and grow.

Safety Precautions

Herbs and herbal medicines have been used effectively throughout human history, and folk remedies are used globally by millions of people every day without incident. This does not mean that every herb is safe or that every herbal remedy is safe for every person. Here are some simple ways to keep yourself safe when using herbal medicines and remedies:

- Start with the gentlest herbs, and take them at the lowest dosage at first. Herbs that are rated safe for infants and children, such as lavender, elderberry, and chamomile, are least likely to cause a negative or harmful reaction. You can find information on child-safe and gentle herbs by asking a professional herbalist in person or online, asking people in your online herbal groups, and researching books at the library. There are many great books (such as *Herbs for Children's Health: How to Make and Use Gentle Herbal Remedies for Soothing Common Ailments* by Rosemary Gladstar) that can help guide you.

- Listen to your body! I cannot stress this enough. Far too often in our modern-day society, we are taught to ignore, and even override, the signals our bodies give us. Don't do this when you take an herbal remedy. If you notice sudden-onset headaches, nausea, itchiness, or any negative reaction after taking an herb (especially if it happens consistently when using a specific herb or herb blend), discontinue using it right away. There are so many herbs to choose from, and not every herb is the right fit for every person. Best to be safe.

- If you have prescription medications or take over-the-counter (OTC) medications regularly, *always* be aware of potential herb and drug reactions. Not every herb/drug combination is seriously dangerous, but some can be, especially if they have similar purposes. For example, if you take medication that lowers blood pressure, you do not want to take an herb that does the same. This could lead to dangerously low blood pressure. However, it's more common for the drug and herb to interact in ways that are merely inconvenient. Let's say you're using an herb that stimulates the body while also taking a drug to aid with sleep—they may cancel each other out (or you may be in for a wakeful night).

- Anyone taking prescription medication should be in communication with their healthcare provider. While some allopathic doctors are well-versed in and respectful of herbal medicine, many are not. You must be prepared to advocate for yourself and for your choice to rely on herbal remedies alongside allopathic medications. Be willing to take notes, ask questions about potentially harmful drug/herb interactions, and do your own research. And if your allopathic medical team is unwilling to work with you on your herbal medicine journey, consider finding another care provider who will. Your healthcare experience should be a collaborative effort.

- Be aware of any potential allergic reactions and side effects of the herbs you are ingesting.

- *Always* label your herbal remedies! List the herbal ingredients (in order from highest amount to lowest), the date the remedy was made, when it should be used by, and instructions on dosage.

Essential Tools and Equipment

Here are the supplies I recommend having on hand to craft your herbal medicines and folk remedies with ease:

Jars, specifically glass mason jars and lids. These are easy to find, not too expensive, and simple to sanitize and store. I suggest buying a variety of sizes. My most-used sizes are 8-ounce, 16-ounce, and 32-ounce jars.

Amber glass tincture bottles with or without droppers. These are perfect for tinctures and small-batch syrups. The amber glass protects the contents from light, which keeps it from degrading and losing potency. The dropper

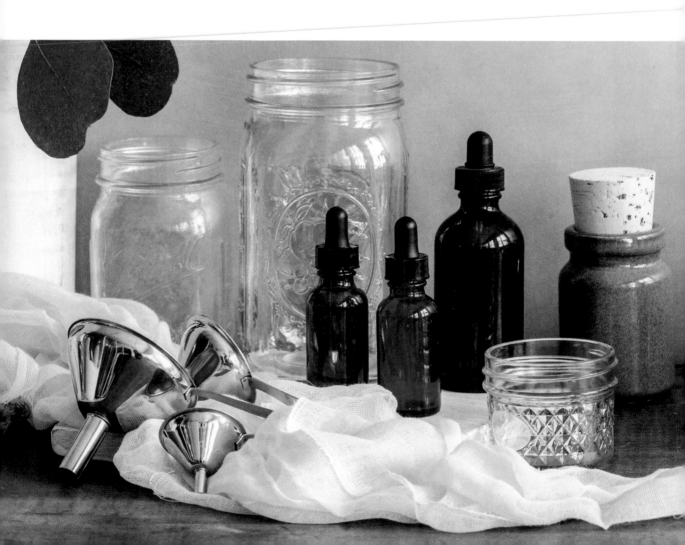

makes it easy to administer the herbal remedy. Dropper bottles typically come in ¼-ounce, ½-ounce, and 1-, 2-, and 4-ounce sizes. Twist-cap bottles come in the same sizes as the dropper bottles and also come in 8- and 16-ounce bottles. I usually bottle part of a tincture in a 2-ounce dropper bottle and store the remainder in bottles with twist caps. Twist caps seal the bottles more tightly, and the alcohol fumes in tinctures can cause the rubber in dropper caps to degrade over time. For spray bottles, I use 4-ounce misters most often.

Food-grade, silicone spatulas in a variety of sizes. These are great for getting the last bits of herbal remedies out of containers.

Funnels. These are a must for getting extracts, syrups, and powders into narrow-mouthed bottles. Canning funnels are great as are basic kitchen funnels. Grab a funnel set with multiple sizes at any store that sells cooking supplies. I prefer using silicone funnels as they do not slip in the opening of the bottles the way hard plastic and stainless-steel funnels tend to do.

Strainers. I suggest using fine-mesh stainless steel, since it holds up to repeated use and most plant matter can't sneak through the fine mesh into your final product. Having a variety of sizes will make it easier to get the medicine into the containers.

Filters. Unbleached paper coffee filters and muslin tea bag filters work for keeping herbal particulate out of your end product. I personally prefer paper filters, as they are compostable and accessible nearly everywhere; I find that cloth tea bags tend to collect plant matter in the seams. Both, though, are wonderful, sustainable options for herbal medicine crafting.

Cheesecloth. I have cheesecloth on hand for when the herb and plant particulate in my remedies is too small and gets through the fine-mesh filter. The remedy can easily filter through the cheesecloth, which catches the herb and plant material. This remaining material can then be composted.

Small coffee grinder. This appliance is a must to help break down plant material into fine powders. Don't use your herb grinder for coffee, as this will contaminate your end product; buy one specifically for your herbal medicine practice.

Mixing bowls and measuring utensils. I use stainless-steel mixing bowls because I often place my bowl directly on my scale, and the stainless-steel bowls are light and easy to maneuver. I use glass measuring cups for my larger batches and have a 1-cup, 2-cup, and 4-cup set (purchased from Target on sale) that I use constantly. For smaller measuring cups and

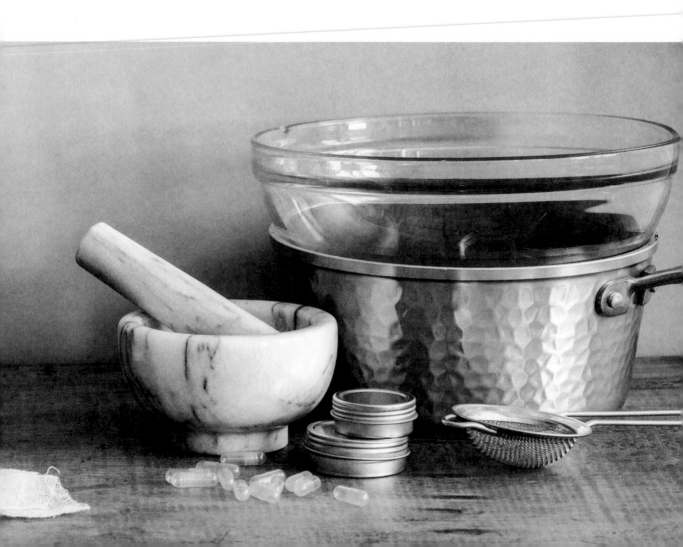

spoons, I use simple stainless-steel sets that you can get from the baking section of nearly any store.

A good kitchen scale. I prefer using a digital scale, since it is calibrated to very small weights and gives more accurate measurements than a weighted scale. You can find a good basic digital scale for less than $20 at Target and on Amazon (and at other suppliers) with a quick search online.

Digital candy thermometer. This tool is useful when you are heating oils and extracts as well as when you need to cook off the alcohol in glycerites.

Food dehydrator. If you have access to a food dehydrator, yay! But if you don't, no biggie. I find that a multi-size set of steel cookie sheets works like a charm for drying herbs.

Double boiler. To set this up, all you need is a small saucepan filled one third of the way with water, with a glass bowl set on top of it. The bowl should not touch the water.

Mortar and pestle. This is a grinding tool used for making both culinary and medicinal herbal preparations. Mortars and pestles come in a variety of sizes and materials, such as wood, stone, marble, granite, and ceramic. The most traditional is stone. Much like cast iron, your mortar and pestle will need to be seasoned if it is made of stone or wood to make sure that the porous surfaces do not release any particulate into your end product.

Garlic press. A garlic press is a metal kitchen tool meant for crushing garlic into a fine paste. It can be used to crack or crush other food and herb materials to prepare them for use.

Helpful Ingredients

Alongside your herbs and plant materials, you may need to find additional ingredients to craft your folk remedies and herbal medicines. Here are some of the common ones:

Food-grade alcohol. Different percentages of alcohol work best to extract different herbs. Most home remedies are crafted using 80-proof alcohol. (You can use potato vodka if you have a gluten sensitivity or intolerance.)

Glycerin. This is a sweet-tasting, mostly clear liquid used for alcohol-free extracts. Glycerins are made from animal fats or vegetable fats. If you have a preference, be sure to read the labels or ask the supplier for clarity.

Empty capsules. Encapsulated herbs are a quick and easy way to ingest herbal remedies. The capsules are manufactured from both animal by-products (gelatin) and all-plant material (tapioca) options.

Plant oils. Almond, apricot, coconut, grapeseed, and olive oils are commonly used when making herbal extracts in an oil base. Other fats, such as lard and butter, may also be needed.

Waxes. Types including beeswax and candelilla wax, which can help create salves and balms.

Carrier oils. These neutral oils are used to dilute herbal blends and essential oils so they absorb more readily into the skin and are easier to spread topically.

- *Beeswax pellets or pastilles.* When using beeswax, I prefer pellets and pastilles to the solid pack for several reasons: They are easier to measure, they melt more quickly, and they're easier to use. It's hard to scrape beeswax from solid blocks, and I don't want to melt the solid block every time I need beeswax.

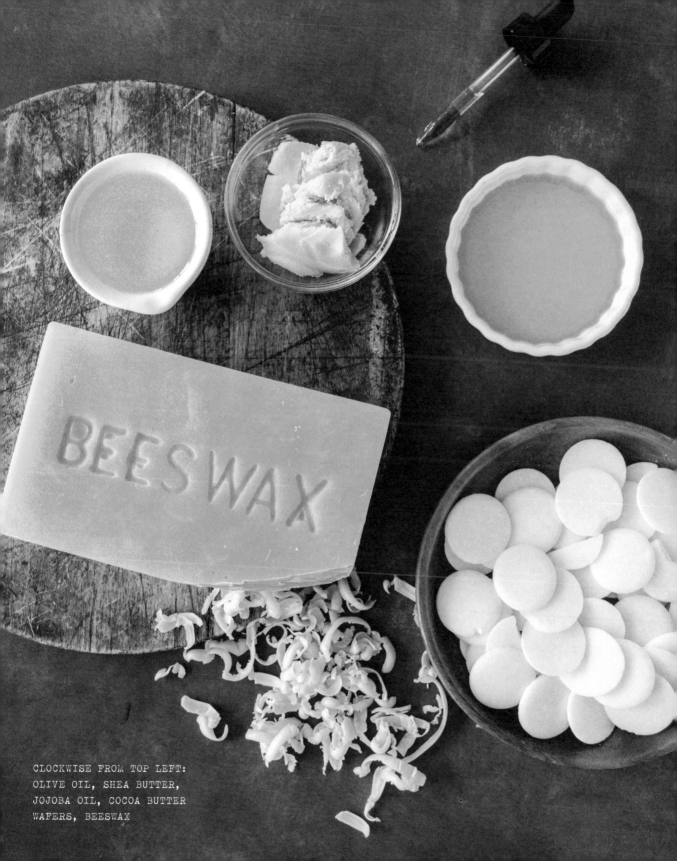

CLOCKWISE FROM TOP LEFT:
OLIVE OIL, SHEA BUTTER,
JOJOBA OIL, COCOA BUTTER
WAFERS, BEESWAX

- *Cocoa butter (unrefined/wafer).* Cocoa butter is an edible fat that is extracted from the cacao bean and comes from the Theobroma cacao tree, which grows in the tropical rainforest regions of Central and South America. It can be used in food products as well as to make body products. Its high levels of fatty acids mean it can help moisturize and nourish the skin while the vitamins and minerals in cocoa butter can help improve and maintain skin's elasticity.

- *Extra-virgin olive oil.* Olive trees are grown globally in the Mediterranean region, North Africa, South America, North America, Australia, and the Middle East. Extra-virgin olive oil is extracted from fresh olives in the first pressing, so the oil is unadulterated and uncontaminated. It is an edible oil that is high in antioxidants and healthy fats. The oil is often incorporated into massage oil and body product blends, as it is soothing to the skin, has a high absorption rate, and is gentle enough for infants, children, and people with sensitive skin.

- *Jojoba oil.* This oil is extracted from the seeds of the jojoba tree. It is indigenous to the Sonoran Desert in North America. Jojoba oil is an unsaturated liquid wax. It is used to ease skin conditions such as eczema and has anti-inflammatory effects on the skin. Its healing properties make it a top choice for healing remedies for hair and skin.

- *Shea butter.* Shea butter comes from the nuts of karite trees, which are indigenous to the Sahel region (an area that extends from East to West Africa and includes Guinea, Senegal, Uganda, and South Sudan). Shea butter contains multiple types of fatty acids, including linoleic, oleic, palmitic, and stearic, which means it acts as a protective barrier for the skin while also moisturizing the skin. Given that the livelihood of traditional Ghanian shea butter crafters is being hampered by large-scale industrial use, I urge you to source your shea butter from traditional suppliers or companies who have a certified fair trade relationship with traditional shea crafters.

Food Ingredients

Many food allies can be added to herbal remedies. Not only do these ingredients complement the medicinal properties of herbal allies, but they bring their own healing properties to the table to create something that is nourishing, delicious, and able to help you heal. Here are some common foods that can be used to boost your medicinal remedies:

Bulb green onions. A bulb green onion is a green onion that has been permitted to grow a little longer, so that instead of a white tip you have a lovely little spring onion at the end of your green. Best of both worlds, really!

Carrots. These vegetables are part of nearly every household's food intake. And I am sure that many of you have heard how carrots can help improve vision and eye health. But carrots can do much more than that. Coming in a rainbow of colors, carrots can help lower blood pressure, improve heart health (red carrots have lycopene), decrease instances of constipation, help keep blood sugar levels stabilized in people with diabetes, offer enough calcium to help keep bones healthy, and boost your immune system.

Cilantro. Not just a flavorful addition to soups and salsas, cilantro has numerous healing properties that make it a wonderful addition to food-based medicinal remedies. Among its many health properties, cilantro helps remove heavy metals from the body, has anticancer properties, works to reduce pain and inflammation in the body, and has natural antifungal properties.

Garlic. Strong in aroma and flavor, garlic is known not only as a culinary must-have but also for its medicinal properties. Among its many abilities, garlic is antioxidant, anti-inflammatory, has fat-lowering properties, helps lower blood pressure, and has been shown to help with diabetes.

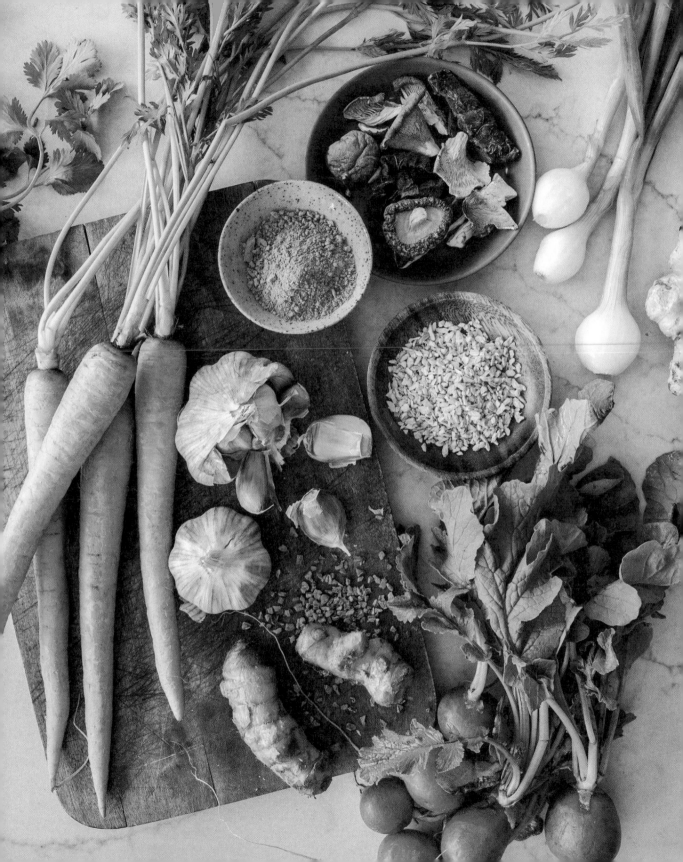

Onions. Onions are inexpensive, extremely accessible, and have a multitude of culinary uses. They have a long history as folk remedies for easing chest congestion and eliminating cold symptoms (putting onion on your feet is a traditional cold and flu remedy, and placing onions in a bowl near the bed are said to stop a cough). In addition, onions are high in vitamin C, have anticancer and antioxidative properties, and are good for helping regulate blood pressure.

Raw apple cider vinegar. This liquid is a naturally occurring probiotic that helps support the immune system and improve gut health. It has antioxidative properties and is said to help lower blood sugar levels, lower cholesterol, and help prevent the growth of harmful bacteria with its antibacterial properties. It is also a good source of potassium, phosphorus, magnesium, and calcium. It can be purchased at most health food stores, but it can also be made easily using apple scraps, honey or sugar, water, and time and patience.

Raw honey (local and organic if possible). I know not everyone has access to raw local honey, but if you do, buy it. It is pricier than its grocery store counterpart, but the benefits outweigh the cost. Raw local honey is naturally antimicrobial and helps the body build resistance to seasonal allergies (due to the fact that the bees are using local pollens). It is also antiseptic and anti-inflammatory. Uncontaminated honey has a forever shelf life (no kidding). Since it is unprocessed, you are getting vitamins and trace minerals (like ascorbic acid, magnesium, potassium, and zinc) while staying away from chemicals.

Dosages and Protocols

Herbal medicines and folk remedies affect the body and impact systems differently than allopathic medications and pharmaceuticals. Some herbal remedies make an immediate and noticeable impact, whereas others have a cumulative effect over a period of weeks or months. Likewise, taking an herbal remedy made from a single herb will have a different dosage than an herb formula crafted from multiple combined herbs.

Dosage Recommendations

Learning the art of crafting herbal medicine goes hand in hand with learning how to properly dose your remedies. Improper dosing can lead to a very dissatisfying herbal experience. Taking too high a dose can leave you feeling unwell; taking too small a dose can leave you feeling as if nothing is happening at all. And taking the remedy inconsistently, or with bad timing, can leave you feeling like you are up and down and out of sorts.

Herbal dosage depends on the way in which the herbal remedy is being delivered. A powdered or loose-leaf herb will have a different impact, and need different dosage measurements, than a liquid herb. Herbal remedies can be dosed in multiple ways and volumes, from single drops of extracts and tinctures to multiple tablespoons to cups and more.

When dosing powders or loose-leaf herbal remedies, dosage measurements will likely align with teaspoon/tablespoon/cup measurements. When dosing tinctures, the dosing can vary depending on whether the measurement is done in drops, dropperfuls, milliliters, a pump, a spray, a teaspoon, or a tablespoon. This can get even more confusing depending on the size of the dropper, pump, or spray, the thickness of the tincture or extract, and the base liquid the herb is in—such as alcohol, glycerin, or an alcohol/water mix. On average, if you use the dropper method, a single dropper will hold between 20 and 30 drops, or about 1 mL. A ¼ teaspoon of tincture is about

1.2 mL, so if a remedy calls for 1 dropperful and you don't have a dropper, use ¼ teaspoon instead. A teaspoon of tincture will be approximately 5 mL.

Dosage is often based on age (adult or child), body weight, acuteness of symptoms, and the particular herb or herbal blends involved. Traditional dose suggestions on ready-made tinctures, syrups, and extracts generally base the dosage on a mid-size adult (130 to 150 pounds). I suggest decreasing the dosage for smaller adults and for people more sensitive to herbal remedies, and increasing the dosage for larger adults and people who have a higher tolerance for herbal remedies.

Also, dosing differs depending on what type of illness you are working to treat. An illness might be acute, coming on suddenly and with intensity. It might be subacute, lingering past the acute stage but not quite a chronic condition. It might be chronic, where it is persistent or long-lasting in its symptoms and effect on health. Or it might be degenerative, where it begins to cause noticeable loss of healthy function in the body over the long term.

For acute illness, a functional general rule is to take small doses more frequently, think every 15 minutes to every 2 to 3 hours for about 2 to 3 days, or as the symptoms persist. Once the symptoms and illness have passed, continue dosage every 3 to 4 hours for the next 7 to 10 days. This helps bolster the system as it moves back into a healthy state.

For subacute illness, a good suggested dosage is every 2 to 3 hours.

Chronic illnesses often call for low-dosage management, 1 to 3 times a day. Be aware that when treating chronic illness, "new" symptoms may surface as more intense or noticeable symptoms improve or go away. These symptoms may have been present the entire time, and herbal remedy treatments may need to shift to begin addressing them. (Think of it like this: If I broke my arm and it was also scraped and bleeding, the pain of the break would likely override my notice of the pain of the scrapes and superficial injuries. As the break is dealt with and that pain subsides, my attention will shift to the other issues. The scrapes were there the entire time, but they were overridden by the more severe issue of the broken bone.)

For degenerative illness, dosages are the same as for chronic illness but with a longer timeline for symptoms improving. The remedies in this book that address degenerative illness and chronic illness have dosage suggestions to help guide you.

Practical Protocols

It can often be difficult know whether an herbal remedy is working. Here are some ways to gauge efficacy:

- Do you feel *any* changes? If not, you might need to increase the dosage. If you still have no effects, this herb may not be the right one for you.

- Do you feel unpleasant effects? Nausea, dizziness, sudden-onset headaches, or other negative body signals may be a sign that you need to lower the dosage or discontinue the herbal remedy.

- If the original herb does not have an effect, or has a negative effect, try another herb or set of herbs with similar properties.

Checking Contraindications

Contraindications are specific situations in which a medicine, procedure, or surgery should not be used because it may be harmful. I know it is not always possible to check in with an allopathic doctor or healthcare provider when seeking information on whether an herb or herbal remedy may contraindicate with a medication you take; another way to check on potential drug/herb safety issues is to speak with a well-versed herbalist. There are also books you can consult, such as *Herbal Contraindications and Drug Interactions: Plus Herbal Adjuncts with Medicines,* American Herbal Products Association's *Botanical Safety Handbook,* and *Herb, Nutrient, and Drug Interactions: Clinical Implications and Therapeutic Strategi*es, many of which can be borrowed from your local library.

Substituting Herbal Allies

It is the work of every herbal practitioner to protect our plant allies and the environments in which they grow. Sadly, as herbal medicine and folk remedies are seeing a much-needed rebirth, many people new to herbal medicine get overexcited with their foraging and harvesting behaviors. This has led to the near extinction and endangerment of many commonly used herbs, such as ginseng and slippery elm. Learning to protect these at-risk, endangered herbal allies is a must.

One way we can do this is to find and work with non-endangered plants and herbs that are interchangeable. There are many herbs that have the same or similar effects on the human body. For example, endangered slippery elm and safely accessible marshmallow root can be used interchangeably.

In the event there is no herbal substitute for an at-risk herb, I suggest sourcing the endangered herb in very small amounts (only what is needed for the immediate recipe) from a reputable, sustainable herb company or a trusted local herb shop.

You can also consider growing rare herbs yourself or connecting with local herb growers in your area who work with endangered herbs. An excellent place to start would be your local herb exchange or herbal guild, if you have access to one in your area.

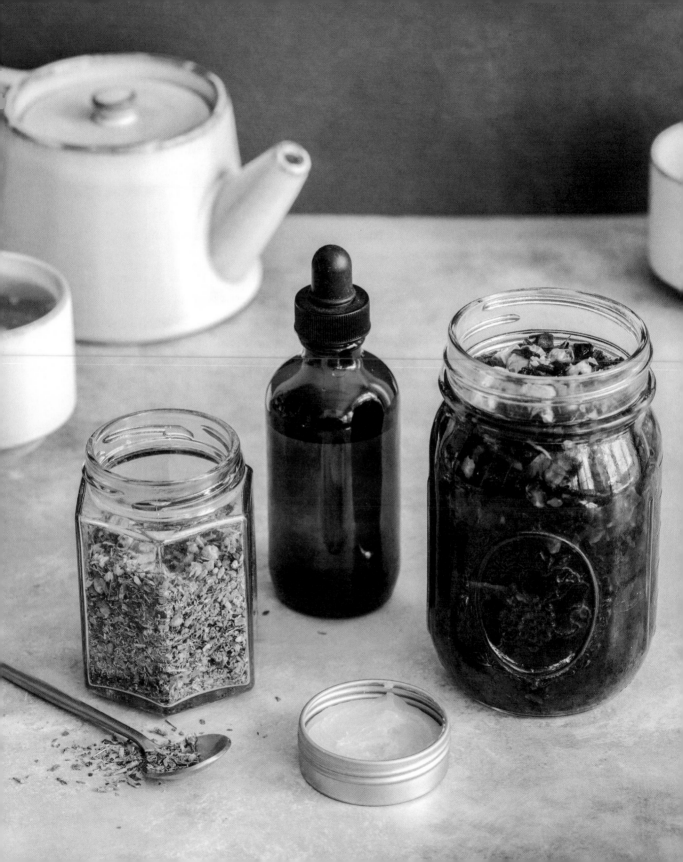

3

HERBAL PREPARATIONS
AND APPLICATIONS

Herb crafting is an art. It is the art of picking the right plant, root, leaf, or herb for the task at hand. Whether you are putting together a single-plant tea or concocting an elaborate salve, the process of preparing the herbs and the ways in which you wish to work with them is critically important. As you move through this chapter, you will learn more about preparing herbal remedies as well as the properties of common herbal preparations.

Teas

What is a tea? Well, my first answer is that tea is Liquid Love in a mug! But tea is so much more than just a cozy hot beverage to sip on a cold winter's day or a cool and soothing friend to savor in summer's heat. Tea is truly special. In many countries around the world, "taking tea" is a daily practice. And in many places, imbibing tea is a form of art and a Sacred ritual. And on top of all these simple glories, tea is an "everyday magic" way of bringing healing herbs into the body.

Before we jump into the art of tea crafting, I want to share a secret with you: Herbal teas are not really tea at all. In fact, they are what is called an herbal tisane. "True" tea comes from a single plant called *Camellia sinensis*. You may be quite familiar with true teas, and may even drink them regularly. Known commonly as black tea, white tea, green tea, pu-erh, and oolong, these beverages are often used to boost energy because of their caffeine content. And though these mighty teas can have a good effect on your health, they are not generally what is being referenced when crafting an herbal tea. That said, they can *absolutely* be a part of a healing tea blend or as a stand-alone tea beverage in your healing tea remedies apothecary. Tea has become the umbrella term for herbal tisanes, true teas, and, honestly, any dried plant, herb, and dried fruit combination that people steep in hot water and drink.

As herbal remedies go, teas provide one of the most affordable and accessible ways to work with herbs. Tea crafting doesn't require much more than herb allies, hot water, and a container in which to brew. On average, you will use 1 to 2 tablespoons of herbal tea blend for every 1 cup of water you use. Loose-leaf tea bags, tea balls, and or loose-leaf strainers are also handy tools to have on hand for steeping loose-leaf teas.

You will need to be mindful with your water. While hardier plant parts can hold up to just-boiled water, I do not suggest pouring just-boiled water onto your tea leaves and flowers. Leaves and flowers contain powerful medicine but prefer a slightly gentler touch. Rather than immediately dousing them in boiling water, let the water settle for a minute or two before pouring it onto your herbs of choice. When working with slightly denser root and rhizome plant allies, such as ginger and turmeric, use just-boiled water and a long steep as well, and/or simmer them directly in the water for up to 15 minutes—whichever is called for in the recipe or for that particular plant or herb ally. Using the correct water temperature gives you full access to the medicinal properties in these plants!

Tea as an herbal remedy leaves wiggle room for dosage. For teas crafted from gentler herbs and other plant allies, such as a ginger-berry blend, a person could safely drink one 8-ounce cup every couple of hours. I suggest using more caution when working with herbal allies and herbal tea remedies that contain stronger herbs, such as our nervine plant relatives, valerian, or poppy. Both ease tension in the nervous system, which is wonderful, but can create extreme drowsiness or cause illness if too much is ingested at once.

There are many ways to store your herbal tea remedies once you have crafted them. Tea tins are a popular, inexpensive, and lightweight option for keeping herbs fresh and dry between uses. My personal favorite way to store tea blends is in glass mason jars with tight-fitting lids. There is just something magical about being able to see all the beautiful herbal medicine blends in their jars. Looking at the bright flowers and vibrant leaves displayed happily on my shelves brings my heart a ridiculous amount of joy! A properly stored tea can last one to two years (though if you're a tea lover like me, they won't last that long).

The main upsides of crafting herbal remedies into teas are that they are easy to make, inexpensive, and last for a long time. Plus, teas can also be used to bring comfort and ease when facing ailments of the soul; a good cup of tea can do as much to fix a bad mood as it can to ease a bad tummy. One of the downsides of teas is that they are sometimes a more diluted form of herbal medicine, and so it may take longer to ingest healing dosages.

As with any herb allies, be sure to purchase from sustainable, reputable retailers. If you have the good fortune to have local herb shops, support

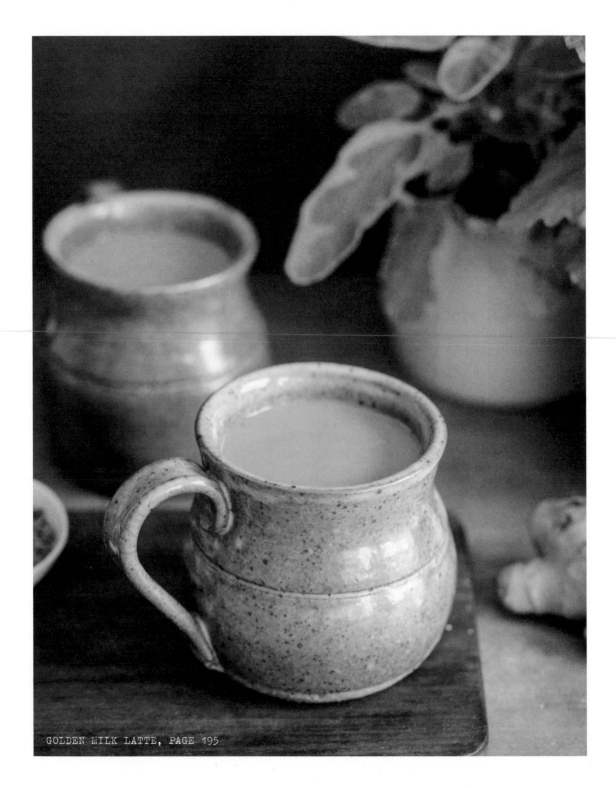

GOLDEN MILK LATTE, PAGE 195

HERBAL MEDICINE FOR MODERN LIFE

them! They are not only purveyors of wonderful herbs, but fonts of knowledge well worth supporting. If you wish to work with an herb that is deeply connected to any specific culture, please find herbalists from that culture, support them, and honor their knowledge. And as I mentioned earlier, if a recipe calls for an endangered plant, seek out an alternative that offers the same properties as the at-risk herb without causing harm to our plant relatives.

Infusions and Decoctions

If you are new to herbal remedies, you may not have ever heard the terms "infusion" and "decoction." And even if you've heard them, you may not know what they mean or how they are relevant to your herbal medicine and folk remedies journey.

An herbal infusion, much like a tea, is an extraction of an herbal plant essence into hot or cold water. You can craft your herbal infusions by working with fresh herbs and plant allies as well as dried herbs and plant material. Herbal infusions can be made from the leaves, stems, and petals/flowers of many different herb and plant allies, each unique in its flavors and properties. And while a tea steeps for a short period of time, usually a few minutes, infusions steep for far longer—anywhere from 15 minutes to 4 hours, even up to overnight for some.

Infusions have played a huge role in my life. I have dealt with adrenal fatigue for many years, and since my first run-in with this health issue, I have been supersensitive and aware when my adrenal system needs support and nourishment. When I feel the slightest signs that my adrenal system is getting overloaded, I always lean heavy on nettles to, quite literally, soothe my nerves. For me, a strong infusion feels the most healing, so I have been known to steep my nettles overnight. When I do a long steep like this, I limit myself to smaller doses and, occasionally, will thin out my dose depending on how my body speaks to me. I learned my lesson when I drank too large a long steep and spent the whole day fighting off sleep!

Much like an infusion, a decoction is an extraction of herb and plant materials into water. However, while an infusion relies on herbs and plant materials whose properties can be extracted by long steeping in warm or hot waters, a decoction is usually crafted from hardier parts of the plants. Roots, bark, dried berries, dried peels, and seeds require more sustained exposure to heat to extract their essence and their oils into water. So while an infusion is steeped, a decoction is simmered. You place the herb and plant allies into a pot of water, cover with a lid, and slowly bring them to a simmer. You'll typically simmer for 20 to 45 minutes, depending on the herb and plant allies involved or the medicinal recipe being followed. Always remember to strain the plant material out of your infusions and decoctions so that they do not cause the remedy to go bad. Even a little piece of leaf or root can grow mold, and it's disappointing to lose a remedy over such a simple misstep.

Infusions and decoctions are among the most frequent preparations of my herbal remedies practice. They are potent and easy to craft with few supplies, and even on days when I feel drained I can still drum up the energy to set herbs to steeping or simmering (though on my most tired days, I set a timer to remind myself I have something on the stove.) The only big downside for me is that these remedies have a very short shelf life. Once you have strained and jarred your infusions and/or decoctions, they need to be refrigerated and used within a week.

Tinctures and Extracts

Tinctures are high on my list of powerful ways to take in herbal medicine and folk remedies. They are strong, easy to use, and, thanks to the resurgence of herbal medicine, can be found in many natural food stores as well as online. Although they may take a little longer to concoct, having them in your herbal remedies arsenal is more than worth the investment of time.

Unlike herbal teas, infusions, and decoctions, tinctures do not use water to extract the essence from herb allies. Instead, tinctures are made by placing various parts of the herb and plant materials into alcohol. First you gather the herbs and plant material, making sure they are washed well and chopped into small, coarse pieces. You then place them into a glass mason jar and cover them with alcohol, filling the jar to the top. Seal the jar, then give it a good shake to mix the alcohol with the herbs and plant material. Leave the jar sealed for six weeks or more (the length of time will vary based on the herbs used in the tincture). Don't forget to give the jar a good shake every day or so to make sure all of the plant material is exposed to the alcohol equally.

Crafting an extract is similar to crafting a tincture. The big difference is in the base used. While a tincture uses alcohol, an extract uses glycerin or vinegar (tinctures are best for certain herbs and plant materials that do not break down in glycerin).

Extracts are more potent than tinctures, but tinctures have a longer shelf life than extracts (one year for tinctures versus six months for extracts). Both are powerful forms of herbal medicine to have on hand. In sum, all tinctures are extracts, but not all extracts are tinctures!

Balms

As a holistic wellness practitioner, I use balms in so many ways—in both my personal life and my professional practice—that it is hard to number them all. I have used them to ease my own achy muscles as well as to treat the sore and tight muscles of my clients, in conjunction with massage. I have soothed cracked skin and calmed small injuries. Balms have served me well over the years.

For all of the wonderful benefits of balms, they can take more time to prepare than other herbal remedies. Work on them when you have abundant time and energy, not when you are feeling depleted and in need of rest. Crafting balms can be a fun experience and I absolutely love how my home smells when I am making them for my apothecary.

To craft your balms, you will need a handful of supplies. Gather two glass bowls (one to use with a pot as part of a double boiler), a pot, a fine-mesh strainer, and glass mason jars with lids. You also need your herbs, beeswax, oil, and butter (if you are using any).

To make an herbal oil infusion, place the herbs and oil into the glass bowl and set the bowl above simmering water in the pot. This step can take 15 to 20 minutes, or more, and you need to be sure that the water in the pot does not touch the bottom of, or get into, the bowl. Pour the oil infusion through the strainer into the second bowl and add the beeswax. Place the bowl with the beeswax onto the double boiler for 5 to 15 minutes, or per the recipe, or until the beeswax melts fully. Once everything is melted together, pour the mixture into clean glass mason jars and let sit, uncovered, on the counter to solidify at room temperature. It can take 1 to 2 hours for the balm to become mostly solid. Finally, cover and store. These little jars of love have a shelf life of up to six months.

Other Herbal Preparations

There are a few other herbal preparations I would like to mention before we move on to crafting herbal remedies. Syrups, powders, compresses, sprays, and oxymels as well as herbal medicine–infused foods are all important components of your herbal medicine cabinet. You'll find recipes for all of these preparations in part three of this book!

- Syrups, such as elderberry syrup, are delicious and convenient ways to soothe coughs, colds, allergies, and sore throats.

- Herbal powders can be used in capsules, as part of a morning beverage, as a part of a smoothie, or on oatmeal, and are more concentrated than loose herbs.

- Compresses are cold herbal infusions soaked into a clean cloth and placed onto an affected area to help accelerate the healing process.

- Sprays can be either topical or for internal ingestion, and help soothe injuries and illness.

- Oxymels are herbal medicinals crafted from honey, vinegar, and herbs that can be used in much the same way as a syrup or tincture to ingest herbal medicine. Oxymels should be kept in cool, dry places but do not need to be refrigerated as the honey and vinegar are both natural preservatives.

There are so many ways to work with herbal allies, and with each different style of preparation you will learn and grow as you expand your herbal medicine crafting skills. As you get more comfortable with creating these different remedies, you can get more adventurous with your herbal combinations—and that is where the real fun starts. Experiment, get curious, and make some amazing herbal remedies! In the next section, you will meet some of the many plant and herb allies you will work with, and learn some basic information about each.

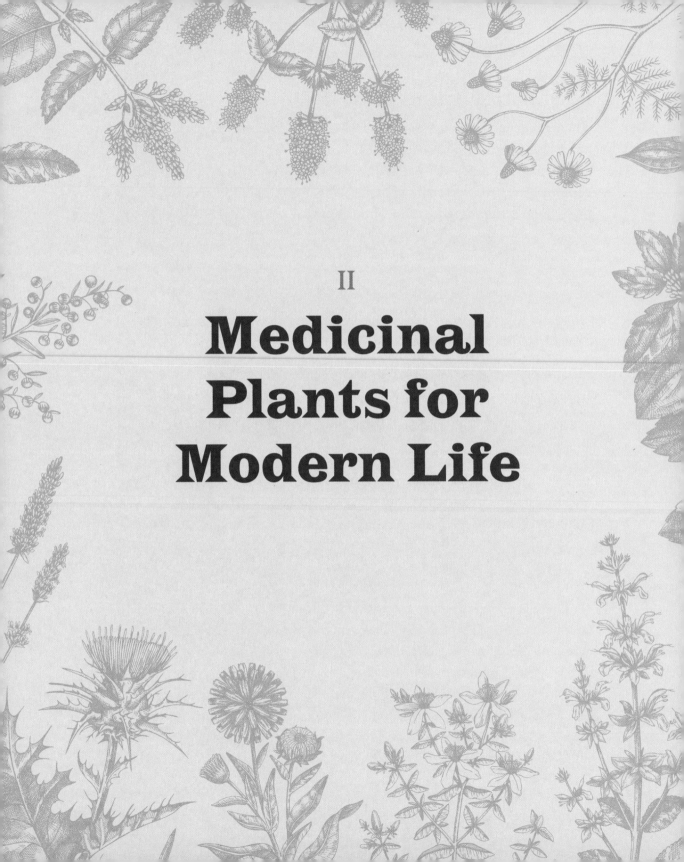

II

Medicinal Plants for Modern Life

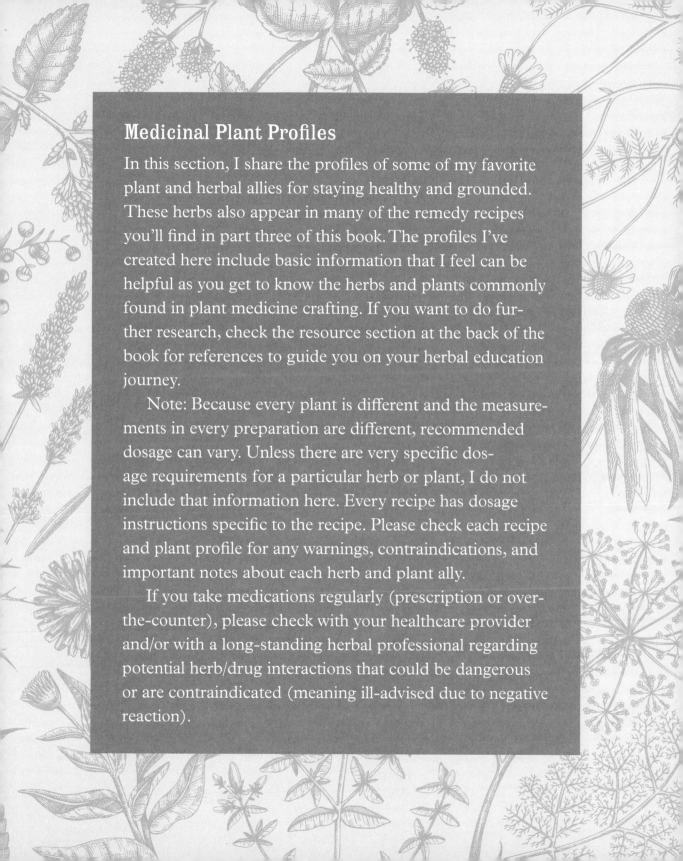

Medicinal Plant Profiles

In this section, I share the profiles of some of my favorite plant and herbal allies for staying healthy and grounded. These herbs also appear in many of the remedy recipes you'll find in part three of this book. The profiles I've created here include basic information that I feel can be helpful as you get to know the herbs and plants commonly found in plant medicine crafting. If you want to do further research, check the resource section at the back of the book for references to guide you on your herbal education journey.

Note: Because every plant is different and the measurements in every preparation are different, recommended dosage can vary. Unless there are very specific dosage requirements for a particular herb or plant, I do not include that information here. Every recipe has dosage instructions specific to the recipe. Please check each recipe and plant profile for any warnings, contraindications, and important notes about each herb and plant ally.

If you take medications regularly (prescription or over-the-counter), please check with your healthcare provider and/or with a long-standing herbal professional regarding potential herb/drug interactions that could be dangerous or are contraindicated (meaning ill-advised due to negative reaction).

Arnica

Arnica montana

Arnica is a bright yellow flower that originated in Europe but has long since naturalized to the mountainous regions of North America. Its prolific blooming season begins in midsummer and continues well into fall. Arnica flowers are best harvested early in the blooming season.

Why I Love This Herb As a retired professional ballet and modern dancer and the mother of six children, I have built a very close relationship with arnica. I used the topical cream often to ease lumps, bumps, and bruises—my kids' and my own. It is a powerful herb ally and a little goes a long way.

Qualities Arnica is warming, drying, relieves pain, helps with high blood pressure, and helps heal wounds.

Plant Family Asteraceae (also known as the daisy plant family)

Medicinal Parts Arnica flowers are the commonly used part, though fresh leaf and root as well as dried leaf are used in tincture preparations.

Ideal for Addressing Arnica works best at addressing inflammation, muscle pain, soreness, and bruising and reduces swelling associated with injury or trauma.

Most Common Preparations Arnica is most commonly used as a topical cream, salve, ointment, or oil.

Important Considerations Though arnica is commonly taken internally as a homeopathic remedy, it can cause gut irritation. It is wise to note that it can be toxic if too much is ingested. Signs of toxic interaction are dizziness, arrhythmia, tachycardia, shaking, and collapse. Arnica is a blood thinner (prevents blood clots from forming), so it should not be taken with other medications or herbs/herbal remedies that do the same, such as aspirin, warfarin, ginger, garlic, or ginseng to name a few. Arnica tincture should not be taken internally by pregnant or nursing people. Do not apply to broken skin. Arnica can cause contact dermatitis for people who have skin sensitivities. Be mindful if you are allergic to plants in the Asteraceae and/or Compositae families, such as daisies, ragweed, dandelions, and chrysanthemums, as arnica could trigger an allergic reaction.

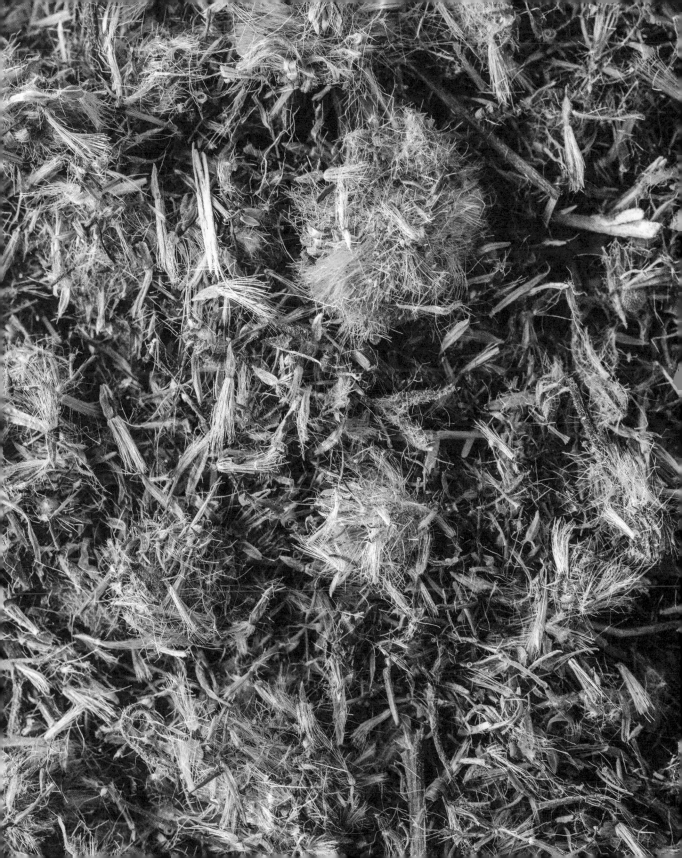

Black Pepper

Piper nigrum

Black pepper is one of the most commonly used, and probably the most readily recognizable, herb across the globe. The distinct, dark, pebble-like peppercorns of black pepper range in color from lightish brown to dark brown, almost black. Black pepper stays freshest and is most aromatic when stored as whole peppercorns and ground fresh for remedies (though the whole peppercorns are also effective).

Why I Love This Herb I literally don't go a meal (let alone a day) without black pepper—either as whole peppercorns or freshly ground pepper—in drinks and meals for myself and my children. It pairs beautifully with nearly every herb, can be both bold and subtle in its flavor, and enables us to use less salt because it accentuates the flavors with which it interacts. And when paired with turmeric, the one-two punch for anti-inflammatory goodness is unmatched.

Qualities Black pepper is warming, antioxidative, anti-inflammatory, improves blood sugar, improves brain function, promotes gut health, and offers pain relief.

Plant Family Piperaceae

Medicinal Parts The peppercorn, which is the dried fruit of the pepper plant

Ideal for Addressing Black pepper is often used in combination with other herbs. When combined with turmeric, black pepper increases turmeric's anti-inflammatory properties by increasing the body's curcumin absorption by 2,000 percent!

Most Common Preparations Black pepper is most commonly used as a spice in foods as well as a complementary herb in herbal remedies.

Important Considerations Eating too much black pepper can cause indigestion, heartburn, and gastrointestinal issues. Inhaling too much pepper into the lungs can be incredibly dangerous and potentially fatal, especially to children. People with allergies to black pepper can have severe respiratory reactions to it.

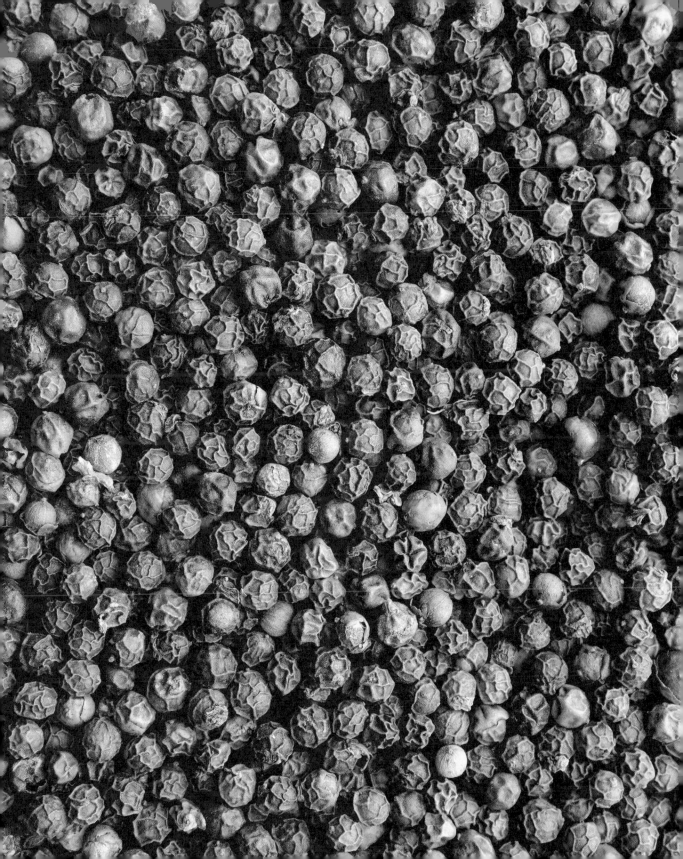

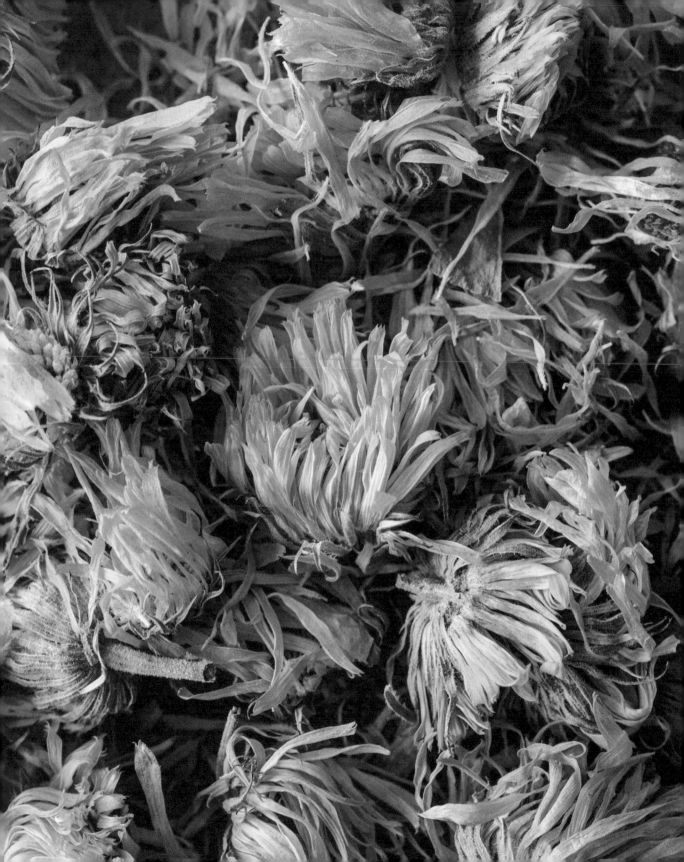

Calendula

Calendula officinalis

Calendula, also known as pot marigold, is a bright, sunny flower that graces many a garden. Native to Southwestern Asia, Western Europe, Micronesia, and the Mediterranean, calendula is prolific and grows nearly anywhere it takes seed. Due to its long growing season and its hardiness, calendula is often found blooming even after the first snowfall, and in some warmer climes it will bloom year-round!

Why I Love This Herb My preferred remedy to make with gentle and versatile calendula is body butter, as I tend to have really dry skin, especially in the winter. Calendula soothes my skin in a way that no other herbs can.

Qualities Calendula is cooling, drying, astringent, and antibacterial. It is also vulnerary (an old herbalism term that means capable of healing wounds or treating illnesses).

Plant Family Asteraceae

Medicinal Parts Flower

Ideal for Addressing Calendula is commonly used as a topical healing aid for dry skin, eczema, bruises, and rashes. It can be taken internally to ease gut inflammation and it's good for those who live with Crohn's disease and gastritis. It also helps with fevers and pain associated with menstruation.

Most Common Preparations Some of the most common preparations for calendula are salves and body butters.

Important Considerations Calendula has no reported toxicity and is safe when working with babies and children. Be mindful, though, if you are allergic to plants in the Asteraceae and/or Compositae families, such as daisies, ragweed, dandelions, and chrysanthemums, as it could trigger an allergic reaction. Calendula is not recommended for internal use during pregnancy, as there is the possibility that it can trigger a miscarriage. This is because it is an emmenagogue and can potentially stimulate uterine contractions. Internal use is also advised against while nursing. Topical applications are still considered safe during pregnancy and while nursing, but avoid the chest area so that nurslings do not unintentionally ingest any salve.

Cardamom

Elettaria cardamomum

Cardamom is an aromatic herbal ally that is actually the fruit of a tropical plant closely related to ginger. I have some ethical concerns around the growing process of cardamom. It is cultivated on plantations in Guatemala and India, and the production and harvesting of cardamom is being affected greatly by intensifying weather events caused by climate change. This, in turn, is causing a shortage in the herb's availability and spiking its prices. When buying cardamom, make sure you are purchasing ethically from a reputable fair trade source or direct from farmers.

Why I Love This Herb Cardamom makes me think of fall and the delicious treats I craft during that time of year. Its scent is immediately calming to me and is one of my go-to herbs for warming seasonal beverages. I like to combine it with cinnamon and nutmeg (two other warming, aromatic herbs) when my stomach feels grumbly.

Qualities Cardamom is warming, drying, carminative (an older herbalism term that means it relieves gas), aromatic (has a strong scent at room temperature), and a respiratory aid.

Plant Family Zingiberaceae

Medicinal Parts Pods, hulls, and powder

Ideal for Addressing Cardamom is used as a digestive aid.

Most Common Preparations Cardamom is most commonly used in its powder form as a culinary herb. In Ayurvedic culinary/medicine practices, the whole pod is used more often, or grated into fresh powder. (Ayurveda is a system of traditional medicine native to India.) Many people do not realize that cardamom also has medicinal properties.

Important Considerations Cardamom is contraindicated, in large doses, for pregnant people and people taking blood thinners. Cardamom is found in many foods, and small amounts of cardamom are classified as safe. If you are pregnant or taking blood thinners and feel concerned, please speak with your healthcare provider.

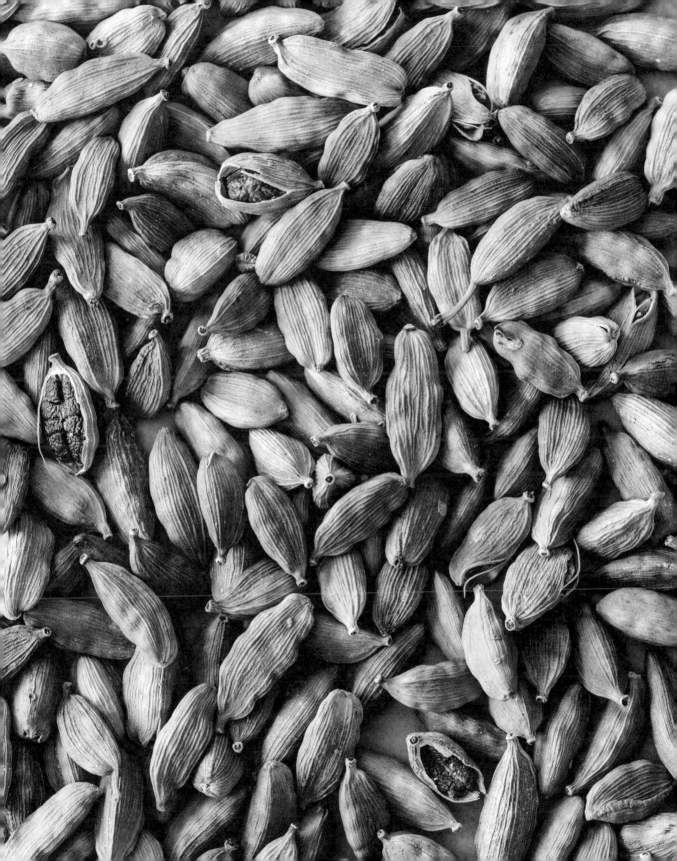

Cayenne Pepper

Capsicum annuum

Cayenne is a global superstar. A culinary spice as well as a medicinal herb, cayenne was known to the Indigenous peoples of North America as far back as 9,000 years ago. With its bright color and moderate to high heat score, cayenne is a great addition to the spice rack and medicine cabinet.

Why I Love This Herb Cayenne pepper adds a hint of color, a bit of heat, and a sharp flavor to everything. It is warming and soothing at the same time. I find it to be exactly what is needed when I am cooking chili and I love the heat it creates in my pain-rub salves.

Qualities Cayenne is warming, drying, a pain reliever, helps relieve gas, can slow and stop bleeding, and acts as a heart tonic and a digestive aid.

Plant Family Solanaceae (nightshade)

Medicinal Parts Only the fruit is edible and/or medicinal. The leaves, stems, and flowers can be toxic.

Ideal for Addressing Cayenne helps with pain relief, offers digestive aid and immune support, stimulates endorphin release, helps with ulcers, and is heart health supportive.

Most Common Preparations Though cayenne is most often used as a culinary spice, one of its main active ingredients, capsaicin, is so renowned for its pain-relieving properties that it is now used as an active ingredient in many commercial pain-relief creams.

Important Considerations Though cayenne is perfectly safe to use, it can cause gastrointestinal distress for some people. Keep it away from eyes, genitals, and the sinus cavity, as it can cause intense burning to these sensitive areas. Internal ingestion is not recommended for people with hemorrhoids.

Chicory

Cichorium intybus

Chicory has bright blue flowers that look bouquet ready, though it is classified as a weed by some. Its large root is popular for roasting and adding an earthy flavor to beverages; its leaves are commonly used in salads. Native to Europe, chicory has become naturalized in North America.

Why I Love This Herb I love to make noncoffee using chicory and dandelion root. It has such a unique flavor and aroma and is quite soothing.

Qualities Chicory is cooling and cleansing for the body. It is an antioxidant, antidiabetic, and prebiotic.

Plant Family Asteraceae

Medicinal Parts Leaves and roots

Ideal for Addressing Chicory promotes healthy digestion, regulates appetite, supports liver function, stimulates bile production, and has been shown to decrease the risk of gastrointestinal illnesses and diseases.

Most Common Preparations Roasted chicory root is used in decoctions, extractions, and infusions. It has become a popular coffee replacement because it has an amazingly tart and slightly bitter flavor without the caffeine or the crash.

Important Considerations Chicory should be avoided by people with irritable bowel syndrome (IBS) and by pregnant and nursing people. If you take medication for diabetes, be aware that chicory has blood sugar–lowering properties that, if taken alongside diabetes medication, can cause blood sugar to drop dangerously low. Chicory stimulates the gallbladder and can aggravate gallstones. Be mindful if you are allergic to plants in the Asteraceae and/or Compositae families, such as daisies, ragweed, dandelions, and chrysanthemums, as it could trigger an allergic reaction.

Cinnamon

Cinnamomum verum

Cinnamon has been used for thousands of years in both traditional Eastern and Western medicine practices. Ceylon cinnamon (a.k.a. *cinnamomum verum*), which comes from Southern India and Sri Lanka, and cassia cinnamon (*cinnamomum cassia*), which comes from China, are the two most commonly used. It is a highly valued ally in both Ayurveda and traditional Chinese medicine for its multiple uses and strong medicinal affinity.

Why I Love This Herb Cinnamon is one of my favorite spices. I take it *every* day, and start most of my mornings with a hot herbal concoction composed of cinnamon with secondary notes of turmeric, nutmeg, black pepper, ginger, pink Himalayan rock salt, and honey, with boiling water poured over it. Divine!

Qualities Cinnamon is warming, drying, and constricting. It has antidiabetic, antiseptic, astringent (shrinks/tightens body tissues), and aromatic properties.

Plant Family Lauraceae (laurels)

Medicinal Parts Inner bark of the tree, as chips, sticks, and powder

Ideal for Addressing Cinnamon is used to lower blood sugar and increase the ability of the pancreas to produce insulin. It stimulates the circulatory system. It is also used to regulate menstrual bleeding for people dealing with heavy blood flow. (This I can attest to 100 percent; it not only regulates the flow but also nearly eliminates the cramps!)

Most Common Preparations Cinnamon is most commonly used as a culinary spice. It is used medicinally in tinctures, teas, glycerites, capsules, and powders.

Important Considerations Cinnamon is an emmenagogue, which means that it can stimulate uterine contractions, so it's best to limit cinnamon to culinary use during pregnancy.

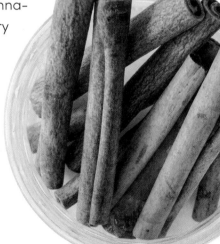

Clove

Syzygium aromaticum

Clove is a strongly aromatic herb cultivated throughout Africa, Asia, and South America. Used in mulling spices, chai blends, and curry seasoning, cloves have long been a culinary powerhouse. But they also have powerful medicinal properties, including soothing nausea, supporting digestion, and helping ease tooth pain.

Why I Love This Herb A little goes a long way with this beautifully intense herb, whether in cooking or for medicinal purposes. Most frequently, I use cloves when dealing with toothaches and oral pain.

Qualities Depending on whom you ask, cloves may be classified as either a cooling spice (in Ayurvedic practices) or a warming spice. They can help calm muscle spasms and relieve pain. They also have antiseptic, anti-inflammatory, antibacterial, antioxidant, astringent (shrinks/tightens body tissues), and antiparasitic properties.

Plant Family Myrtaceae

Medicinal Parts Dried buds

Ideal for Addressing Because of their astringent properties, cloves are used to numb sore gums for teething children as well as to counteract dental pain in adults. They have been used to assist in digestive disruption (namely stomach aches). Cloves have also been used in oils and creams as a numbing agent, which makes them helpful for nerve pain.

Most Common Preparations Cloves are most commonly employed as whole buds or in powder form. They are prepared as infusions, tinctures, and glycerites, and the oil is often applied topically. Clove essential oil, in a diffuser, is also good for aromatherapy.

Important Considerations Do not take clove oil internally without the supervision of a healthcare professional. Clove essential oil is quite strong and can cause skin irritation and a burning sensation if not diluted first.

Comfrey

Symphytum officinale

Comfrey is like a whimsical storybook plant. Its purplish-pink flowers dangle from its stalk under broad leaves as if waiting for small woodland pixies to make hats out of them. It is native to many places in Europe as well as some parts of Asia.

Why I Love This Herb I used to be intimidated by comfrey. To me, it carried such old and witchy energy and I shied away from using it. Now, it fascinates me. It is a soothing herbal first aid tool that has withstood the test of time.

Qualities Comfrey is cooling and moistening. It is astringent (shrinks/tightens body tissues), demulcent (protective to mucous membranes), emollient (softens or soothes skin), and helps heal wounds.

Plant Family Boraginaceae

Medicinal Parts Leaf

Ideal for Addressing Comfrey is used frequently for external skin injuries. It contains allantoin, which stimulates healthy cell growth. When used internally, its ability to coat the lining of the stomach and the intestines makes it a helpful herbal ally for persistent digestive problems.

Most Common Preparations Compresses, poultices, and salves

Important Considerations Comfrey can, potentially, cause liver problems when taken internally. It is still taken internally by some people, while others opt to enjoy it externally only. Comfrey should not be taken by people who are pregnant or nursing, who have liver problems, or who have cancer or tumors.

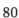

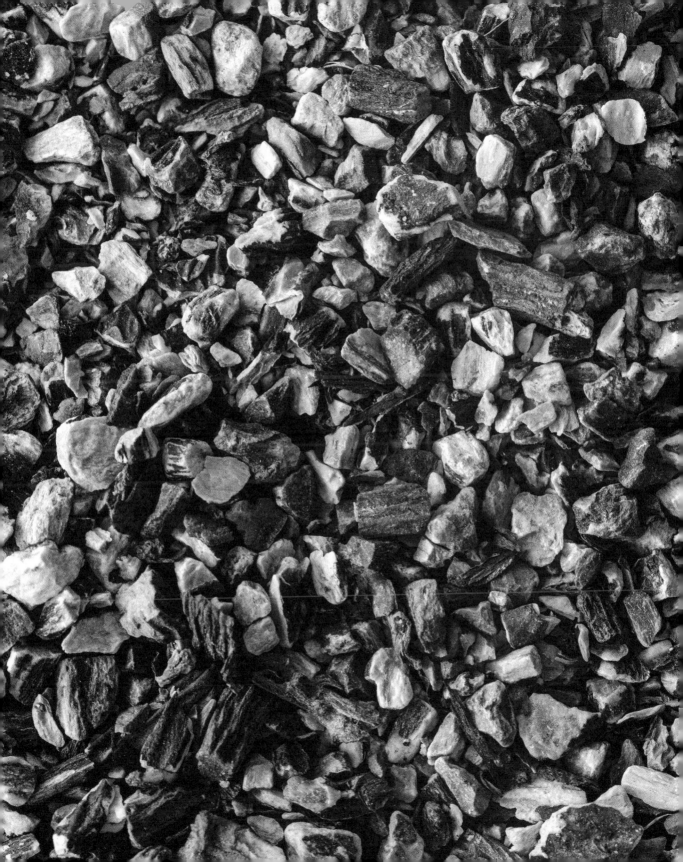

Dandelion

Taraxacum officinale

Dandelion grows the world over. It is both loved and vilified. It has been active throughout history as both medicine and food, with its earliest documented reference back in 659 BCE in the *Tang Materia Medica*. It appears in Ayurveda, traditional Chinese medicine, traditional Indigenous medicine, and in the food practices of various tribes as well as in European medicinal and food practices.

Why I Love This Herb Dandelions are magic. They can grow pretty much anywhere, under nearly any conditions, and still maintain their medicinal capabilities. They are one of the most self-possessed and Zen plants I have borne witness to. I am in awe.

Qualities Dandelion is a cooling and drying herb. It is used as a liver tonic, a diuretic, and aids in digestion due to its nature as a bitter. Dandelion is an aid to metabolism and stimulates bile production.

Plant Family Asteraceae

Medicinal Parts Root, leaf, and flower

Ideal for Addressing Dandelion helps with liver function. It helps support and stimulate the urinary system, the digestive system, and the pancreas.

Most Common Preparations Dandelion root is part of many medicinal preparations. It can be in its raw state or roasted. The young leaves can be in salads and stir-fries as well as teas and tinctures. The flower heads contribute to teas, tinctures, and wines. The young spring leaves are best eaten raw to get the highest nutrient intake. You can make an infusion from the leaf (dried or fresh) as well as decoctions and glycerites.

Important Considerations Dandelions produce a milky-white natural latex that can trigger an allergic rash in some people. Be mindful if you are allergic to plants in the Asteraceae and/or Compositae families, such as daisies, ragweed, and chrysanthemums, as it could trigger an allergic reaction.

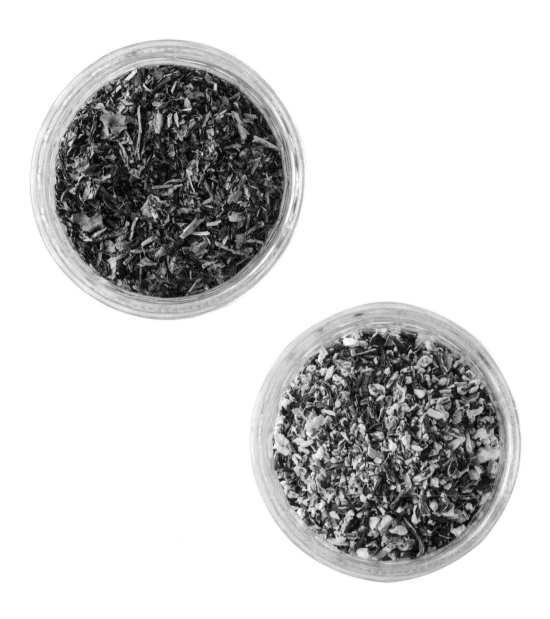

Dulse

Palmaria palmata

Dulse is a red seaweed that is harvested in the North Atlantic along the coasts of North America, Norway, and Ireland. A popular snack, dulse has been eaten in Eastern Canada and Ireland since the twelfth century. It can appear as flakes, powder, in dried sheets, and dried whole plant pieces. As an extract, dulse has been available to help lower blood pressure, improve eyesight, and aid in the improvement of thyroid health.

Why I Love This Herb I love dulse for its light and sweetish flavor as compared to other seaweeds. It is more subtle and mixes well with other seaweeds and works beautifully in herbal remedies.

Qualities Dulse is a cooling, moistening, and nourishing plant ally. It has nutritive properties as well as being an emollient, and it helps the body absorb minerals with ease.

Plant Family Palmariaceae

Medicinal Parts Leaf

Ideal for Addressing Dulse is high in iodine, which can be helpful to people dealing with hypothyroidism. It contains significant levels of potassium and calcium, which help maintain healthy bones. It also assists in lowering blood pressure.

Most Common Preparations Dulse is most commonly known as a food product; it is available in flake and powder form to shake onto food as well as in powder form in capsules. The dried leaves and flakes have been used to create glycerites and tinctures. The leaves have even been used to create a savory sort of tea.

Important Considerations Avoid dulse and other seaweed if you have hyperthyroidism, as the high levels of iodine can be harmful.

Echinacea

Echinacea angustifolia

Echinacea is distinctive; with its beautiful purple-pink petals and dark orange seed cone on a dark reddish stem, it stands out among the daisy family. Echinacea has been overharvested, so be sure to source your supplies ethically rather than using sources that wildcraft their flowers.

Why I Love This Herb Echinacea is a strong immune-supporting herb, one I like to keep in my herbal medicine tool kit at all times.

Qualities Echinacea is cooling and drying. It is antiseptic and antiviral, stimulates the immune system, supports the lymphatic system, and helps support the liver.

Plant Family Asteraceae

Medicinal Parts Seed, flower, leaf, and root

Ideal for Addressing Echinacea is wonderful for addressing illness right at the outset. It has an affinity for relieving upper-respiratory illnesses and works wonderfully to ease sore throats.

Most Common Preparations Echinacea is commonly prepared as a tincture, tea, decoction, or glycerite. It also works well in medicinal syrups and lozenges.

Important Considerations Echinacea is contraindicated for people who have an autoimmune disorder. Be mindful if you are allergic to plants in the Asteraceae and/or Compositae families, such as daisies, ragweed, dandelions, and chrysanthemums, as it could trigger an allergic reaction.

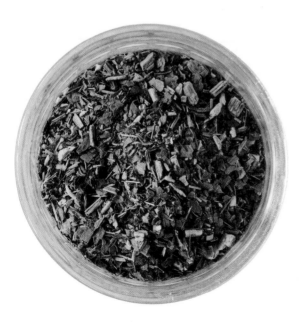

Elecampane

Inula helenium

The elecampane plant looks as if a straw hat and a sunflower had a baby. Its leaves are vibrant yellow and spindly, with a bright orange seed cone in the center. Elecampane grows natively in Southern and Eastern Europe, but thrives prolifically across the globe.

Why I Love This Herb I love how gentle elecampane is. It is a true family herb that can be used with babies and adults alike.

Qualities Elecampane has warming and drying properties. It is a bitter and also an expectorant. It has antiseptic properties and is an antioxidant as well as anti-inflammatory.

Plant Family Asteraceae

Medicinal Parts Root

Ideal for Addressing Elecampane works great with coughs and is often taken to thin mucus. Other benefits are its ability to promote sweating, ease vomiting, and reduce inflammation and swelling. It has also been used to kill bacteria.

Most Common Preparations Elecampane is most commonly found as a tincture though it works well as a tea, a syrup, and a spice.

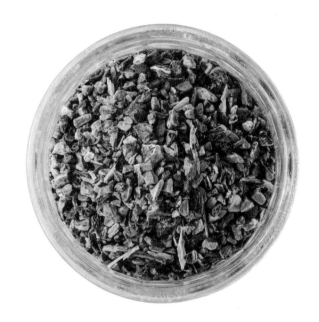

Important Considerations Be mindful if you are allergic to plants in the Asteraceae and/or Compositae families, such as daisies, ragweed, dandelions, and chrysanthemums, as it could trigger an allergic reaction. Large doses can cause nausea, vomiting, diarrhea, and abdominal cramping.

Eucalyptus

Eucalyptus globulus

Eucalyptus plants are majestic, with papery bark of varying shades. The strong aroma of the eucalyptus tree is quite distinct, so you always know when one is near. Native to Australia, eucalyptus was known to the Aboriginal peoples as medicine. Eucalyptus trees are found in so many places in California that they are quite naturalized.

Why I Love This Herb In California, eucalyptus grows everywhere. I like to make bundles out of the branches that fall from the tops of the trees in big winds and hang them in my shower. When the hot steam hits them and they release their oils into the air, it is like being in a steamy herbal sauna. And by foraging the branches blown from the trees, I am practicing ethical wildcrafting while also being safe from potential pesticide exposure.

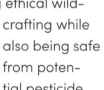

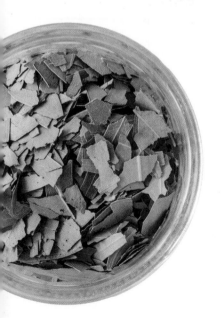

Qualities Eucalyptus is warming and drying. It is antimicrobial, antibacterial, and antifungal.

Plant Family Myrtaceae

Medicinal Parts Leaves and oil

Ideal for Addressing Eucalyptus can help reduce coughs, upper-respiratory congestion, and inflammation associated with upper-respiratory illness. It is also known to reduce muscle and joint pain.

Most Common Preparations Eucalyptus is most commonly prepared as a tincture.

Important Considerations Though eucalyptus is safe for ingestion, small doses must be used and monitored in children to avoid potential toxicity.

Fennel

Foeniculum vulgare

Native to the Mediterranean region, fennel is now cultivated globally. It thrives in temperate zones. It was known as far back as 961 BCE in Spain, and historically has acted as a medicinal for Indigenous tribes in North America, Ayurvedic practitioners, traditional Chinese medicine practitioners, and even the ancient Roman naturalist Pliny the Elder.

Why I Love This Herb While I know the many medicinal benefits of fennel, my favorite part about it is the smell. I like to roll a fennel seed between my fingers, releasing the oils and the sweet, warm smell that only comes from fennel. It smells like licorice candy. When I lived in Northern California, my favorite time of year was when the wild fennel was in bloom and I could walk for blocks taking deep whiffs of the sweet smell.

Qualities A warming and drying herb, fennel is also a galactagogue (boosts production of breast milk).

Plant Family Apiaceae

Medicinal Parts Seeds and essential oil

Ideal for Addressing Fennel seeds relieve bloating. They help ease gas and upset stomach as well as any associated pain from a disrupted digestive system.

Most Common Preparations Commonly made into an infusion for sipping, fennel also works well as a tincture and a glycerite.

Important Considerations Use caution during pregnancy.

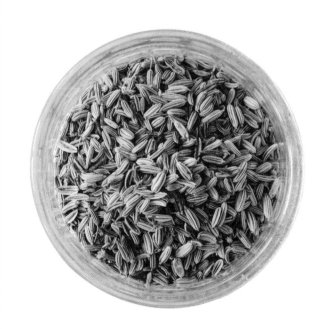

Fenugreek

Trigonella foenum-graecum

Fenugreek originates in North Africa and the countries that border the Eastern Mediterranean. It is an annual herb that has been used for millennia as a culinary herb as well as a medicinal.

Why I Love This Herb Fenugreek holds a special place in my heart for a deeply personal reason. When my youngest was born, she was a micro preemie (only 26 weeks and 3 days). I had no idea if she was going to survive, and my stress and fear stopped my milk production in its tracks. I was devastated and nothing would work. Not goat's rue, not mother's milk blends, nothing. I felt like I was failing. I remember standing in the herbal remedy aisle in tears not sure what to do next. The young herbalist working at the store stopped to chat and when I said I had already tried and failed with fenugreek, he handed me the tincture again and said, "Don't stop taking this until you literally sweat this smell." So I tried again, and as soon as I started to smell like fenugreek, my milk began to flow! Even an old herbalist can learn a new trick.

Qualities Fenugreek is a decongestant and a galactagogue (boosts production of breast milk).

Plant Family Fabaceae

Medicinal Parts Seeds

Ideal for Addressing Fenugreek assists in milk production in nursing people. It has also been used in reducing fevers and regulating blood sugar and cholesterol.

Most Common Preparations Tincture

Important Considerations Fenugreek is contraindicated for pregnancy.

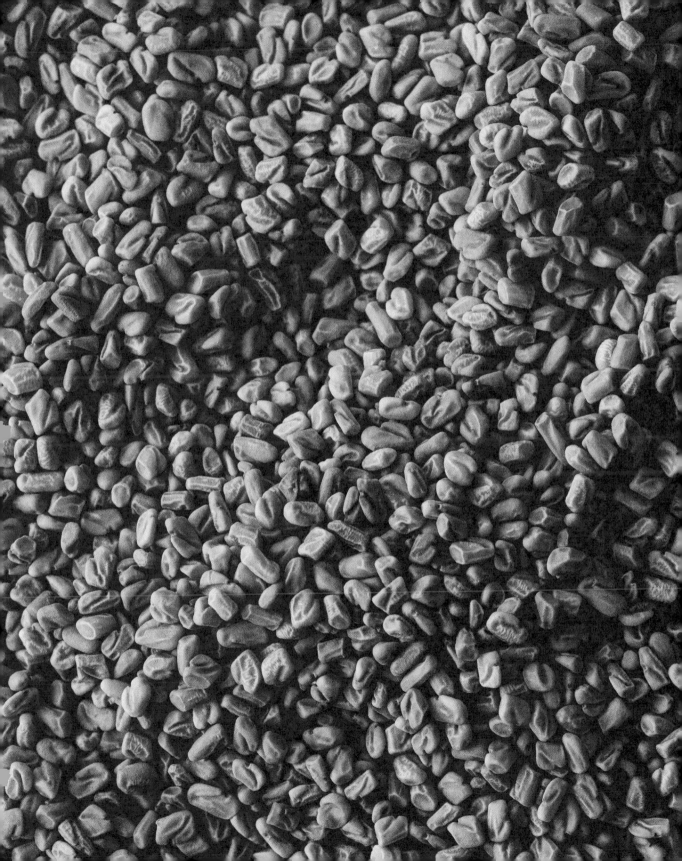

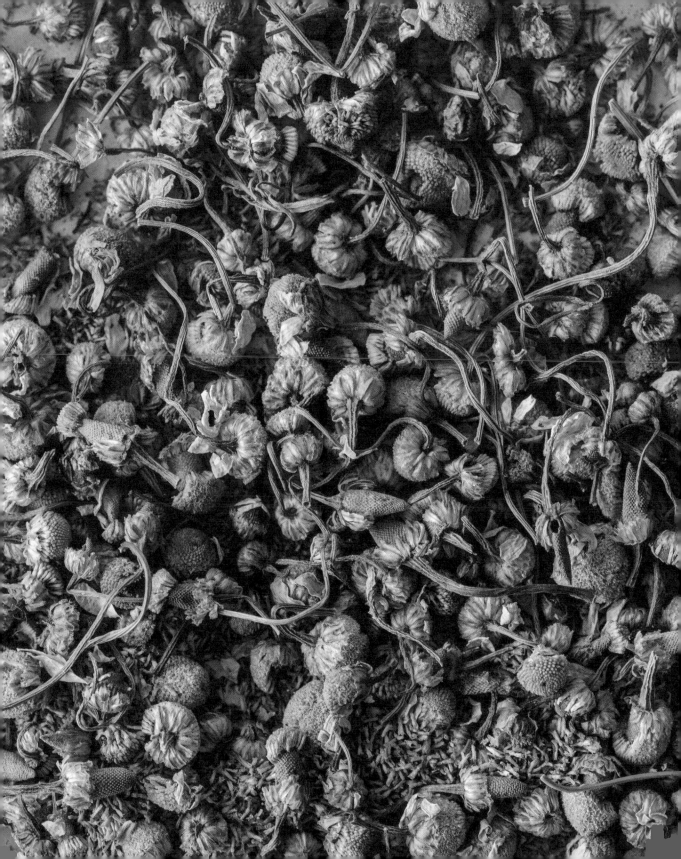

German Chamomile

Chamomilla recutita

German chamomile is a mild sedative. As a nervine, it acts on the nervous system to bring about calm. It is extremely mild and is safe for children. It is known for its distinctive flavor, which is said to taste like apples or pineapples.

Why I Love This Herb German chamomile is a wonderful herb for helping my kids get centered when they feel irritable, out of sorts, or simply can't calm down at the end of the day.

Qualities German chamomile is known to be cooling and relaxing. It is an aromatic, helps calm muscle spasms, and creates a sense of calm.

Plant Family Asteraceae

Medicinal Parts Flower heads

Ideal for Addressing German chamomile is used as a nervine to calm irritability and nervousness. It is also used to ease digestive upset and gassiness.

Most Common Preparations German chamomile is commonly prepared as a tea, but it also makes an excellent tincture and works well in body creams and as an essential oil.

Important Considerations Be mindful if you are allergic to plants in the Asteraceae and/or Compositae families, such as daisies, ragweed, dandelions, and chrysanthemums, as it could trigger an allergic reaction.

Ginger

Zingiber officinale

Ginger is native to Asia and grows throughout the tropics. Though it is often called a root, ginger is, in fact, a rhizome (a continuously growing horizontal underground stem). It is used most often for its culinary properties, but it is highly versatile as both a culinary herb and a medicinal plant ally.

Why I Love This Herb Ginger is my go-to for soothing gut distress. I love the warm and spicy flavor and how well it eases my system. I rely on it for myself and for my children, working with both fresh and dried root and as a powder.

Qualities Ginger is anti-inflammatory, antiviral, helps with nausea, eases and supports digestion, stimulates digestion, and stimulates circulation.

Plant Family Zingiberaceae

Medicinal Parts Rhizome (commonly known as the root)

Ideal for Addressing Ginger is most commonly used to treat digestive complaints. It helps ease nausea, bloating, gas, and abdominal cramping associated with gastrointestinal distress.

Most Common Preparations Ginger is commonly prepared as a tea.

Important Considerations Ginger should not be taken by people who have a bleeding disorder or who take blood thinners.

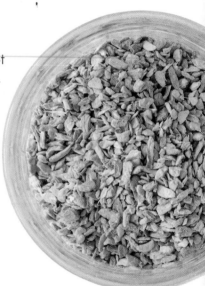

Green Tea

Camellia sinensis

Green tea, and in fact all true teas, come from the same plant. The difference lies in how they are cultivated, when they are picked, and how they are processed afterward. Green tea originated in China. It is said that the discovery of green tea was an accident, occurring when the emperor drank a cup of water that a tea leaf had fallen into. I don't know if this is true, but I am glad we have green tea today.

Why I Love This Herb I love the energy that comes from a good cup of green tea. The bright and earthy flavors, coupled with the strong aroma, create the boost I get from inhaling and drinking green tea.

Qualities Green tea is high in antioxidants. It is a cooling herb. It is also known to reduce inflammation. It supports healthy blood sugar and is good for the heart.

Plant Family Theaceae

Medicinal Parts Leaf

Ideal for Addressing Green tea is used to increase alertness. It is also used as a digestive aid.

Most Common Preparations Green tea is most commonly prepared as a tea.

Important Considerations People taking MAOIs (monoamine oxidase inhibitors) should avoid green tea, as it is contraindicated with the medication.

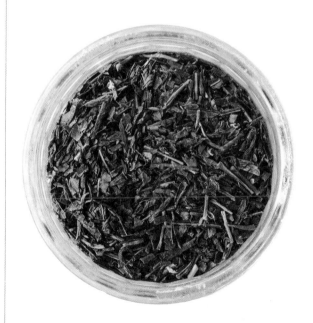

Hibiscus

Hibiscus sabdariffa

This six-foot-tall shrub originated in Africa and Southeast Asia. Its gorgeous, vibrant red flower has been used in Mexican American culture to make the sweet drink agua de Jamaica. Whole flowers can be candied, which gives them the texture of a dehydrated fruit roll.

Why I Love This Herb I grew up drinking agua de Jamaica in the Southern California heat. It was a part of my childhood. I did not know that it was a medicinal herb then; I just knew I loved the flavor. Learning about all the health-supportive abilities of hibiscus have made me love it even more.

Qualities Hibiscus is mildly sedative, supports digestive health, and is a gentle tonic for upper-respiratory health.

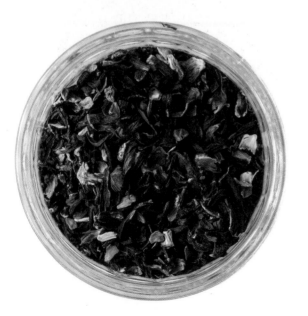

Plant Family Malvaceae

Medicinal Parts Calyx, flowers, leaves

Ideal for Addressing Hibiscus soothes mucous membranes. It is also known for its high level of vitamin C.

Most Common Preparations Hibiscus is most often prepared as a tea. Whether drunk hot or iced, it is a soothing and delicious beverage.

Important Considerations Pregnant people and those who are hypotensive as well as people with high blood pressure who take blood pressure medications, should be careful when ingesting hibiscus as it has been shown to lower blood pressure.

Lavender

Lavandula angustifolia syn. L. officinalis

Lavender is probably one of the most recognized and widely used medicinal herbs by parents (especially of young children). Known for its gentle, baby-safe calming abilities, lavender is in nearly every kind of children's soap, lotion, diffuser oil, and tea. Lavender is native to France and the Western Mediterranean zone, though now it is grown globally and in abundance.

Why I Love This Herb This is one of the first herbs that I introduced to my children, and now to any child who is learning about herbs with me. Its texture and the abundance of tiny flower heads gives little hands the opportunity to explore gently. The smell is calming and children feel compelled to sniff repeatedly, which opens up conversation for their first lesson in aromatics about the power of scent.

Qualities Lavender is antimicrobial, neuroprotective (inhibits damage to brain cells), antidepressant, helps calm muscle spasms, enhances a sense of calm, and relieves anxiety.

Plant Family Lamiaceae

Medicinal Parts Flowers (fresh and dried)

Ideal for Addressing Lavender is a calming herb, and when combined with other sedative herbs, it helps relieve an inability to rest. It has also been shown to ease headaches and migraines. One of the lesser-known properties of lavender is its capacity for easing gas, indigestion, and colic as well as its ability to help heal wounds, sores, and burns.

Most Common Preparations Lavender is most commonly used in essential oil form, though it is also common in teas and tinctures and often used in cooking.

Important Considerations Do not ingest lavender essential oil.

Lemon

Citrus limon

Lemon, notably the dried lemon peel, is a multifaceted plant ally. Not necessarily an herb so much as a culinary food assistant, dried lemon peel holds its own in the medicinals arena. Whether being used in a body product, to complement a sweet or savory food item, or to balance an herbal remedy, lemon is up to the challenge.

Why I Love This Herb While I cannot have lemon (or any citrus) due to a citrus allergy, I love lemon's bright zesty appearance, its uplifting aromatics, and how useful it is as a medicinal.

Qualities Lemon is cooling by its nature. It is antiseptic as well as antimicrobial, antifungal, and antioxidative.

Plant Family Rutaceae

Medicinal Parts Peel

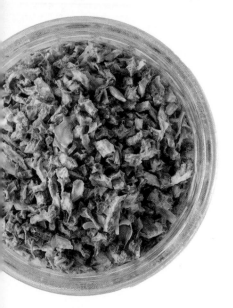

Ideal for Addressing Lemon helps with calcium deposits, gallstones, and digestion. Its scent has been used to increase serotonin and dopamine levels and, in conjunction with other medicinal herbs, it can help ease depression and anxiety.

Most Common Preparations Dried lemon peel is frequently present in tea blends, tinctures, and glycerites.

Important Considerations Do not take dried lemon peel if you have a citrus allergy. Also, there are some studies that show that lemon could negatively interact with hypertension medication. If you take medication for hypertension, speak to your healthcare provider.

Lemon Balm

Melissa officinalis

Lemon balm is native to Southern Europe, Northern Africa, and Western Asia. It is well known for its ability to ease the heart and uplift the mind. Lemon balm's Latin name, *Melissa*, is the Greek word for honeybee. This is because lemon balm attracts bees quite abundantly.

Why I Love This Herb Whenever I think of lemon balm, I can't help but hear the Allman Brothers' song "Melissa." I love lemon balm's delicate lemony aroma, and I find myself crushing leaves just to be able to breathe in the sweet smell. I put lemon balm in many of my remedies, and it has a place of honor in my medicine garden.

Qualities Lemon balm is antiviral, helps calm muscle spasms, and helps relax the mind and body.

Plant Family Lamiaceae

Medicinal Parts Aerial parts

Ideal for Addressing Lemon balm's antiviral properties have been shown to reduce the occurrence of cold sore outbreaks and help clear up any that are present. It calms the nervous system and can aid in alleviating symptoms of depression, anxiety, and unrest. Because of its thyroid-inhibiting effects, lemon balm has been used to decrease thyroid activity in people with hyperthyroidism.

Most Common Preparations Lemon balm is most commonly prepared as a tea or a tincture.

Important Considerations If you have a sensitive thyroid or hypothyroidism, you should not take lemon balm as it inhibits thyroid function.

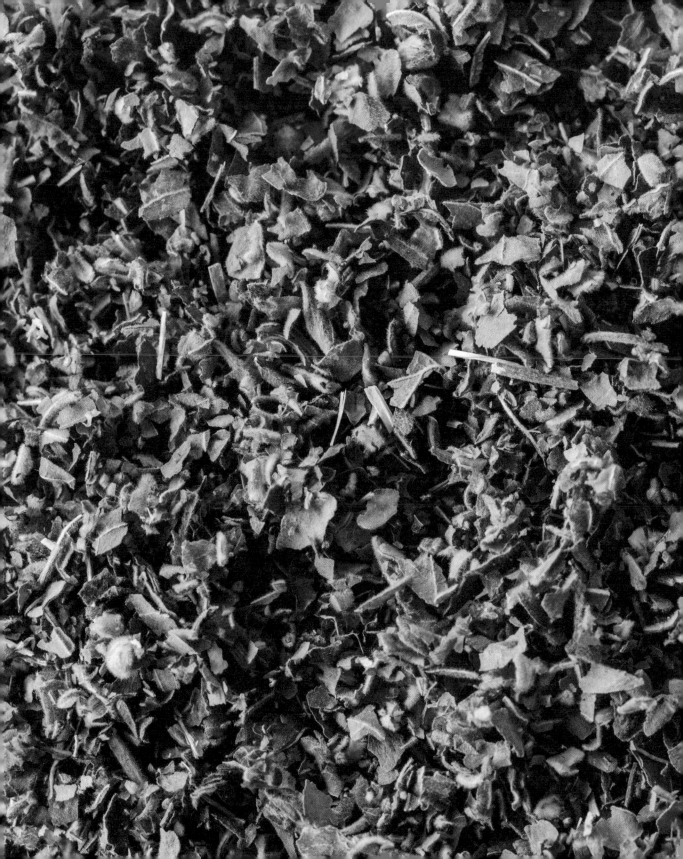

Marshmallow

Althaea officinalis

The marshmallow plant grows to be fairly tall. Reaching up to seven feet, this perennial herb knows how to take up space. It is native to Europe but has become a naturalized plant in North America. Marshmallow loves to grow in marsh zones. It has two harvest seasons: the aerial parts are harvested in summer, and the roots are gathered in fall.

Why I Love This Herb Marshmallow helped me through my early days of long COVID. My digestive tract was all but destroyed, and everything I tried to put into my body made me feel like dying. I drank marshmallow root tea by the quart, alongside pre- and probiotics for months. It took a while, because the impact of COVID on my system was significant, but I was finally able to eat basic, simple foods without feeling intense pain and distension.

Qualities Marshmallow acts as an antioxidant, has mucilaginous (gelatinous, sticky) properties, and antibacterial properties.

Plant Family Malvaceae

Medicinal Parts Flowers, leaves, seeds, and roots

Ideal for Addressing Marshmallow helps protect and soothe the mucous membranes. It is used to counter excessive levels of stomach acid and helps with symptoms of irritable bowel syndrome. It can be used as respiratory support as well, helping calm dry coughs, bronchial inflammation, and the aggravation associated with bronchial asthma.

Most Common Preparations The most common, and optimal, preparation for marshmallow is cold infusion.

Important Considerations If you take any medications, talk to your healthcare provider before taking marshmallow root as it can disrupt the ability of medications to be absorbed. Marshmallow has also shown blood sugar–lowering properties, so it should not be used by people who take diabetes medication.

Mullein

Verbascum thapsus

Mullein is a strong medicinal herb that helps halt viral and bacterial infections. It grows quite well in the wild so can still be wildcrafted (but ethically and with respect to the plant, the environment around the plant, and other potential wildcrafters). Mullein especially likes to grow in uncultivated open fields, alongside the road, and around waste areas, so be mindful when you are foraging for it. Mullein grows to be five to ten feet tall. Its stalk, which grows up the center of the plant, is covered in flowers. Mullein's flowers and leaves are harvested during summer.

Why I Love This Herb This herb is a must in my mother's medicine cabinet. I am fairly prone to ear infections, as are two of my children. I have found that mullein and garlic ear oil work better than repeated use of antibiotics to help relieve the pain, clear the infection, and decrease the frequency of infections. It works so well that my children get the remedy and administer it themselves at the first sign of an ear infection.

Qualities Mullein is an expectorant, antiseptic, antibacterial, antiviral, antioxidant, an emollient (softens or soothes skin), and demulcent (relieves inflammation).

Plant Family Scrophulariaceae

Medicinal Parts Flowers and leaves

Ideal for Addressing Mullein eases coughs and congestion especially when associated with bronchitis. It helps clear airways by bringing up mucus and phlegm in the bronchial tubes and lungs. It also can calm mucous membranes, which soothes any dry or barking cough associated with upper-respiratory aggravation. Mullein oil mixed with garlic oil is often used to relieve ear infections.

Most Common Preparations Mullein is most often prepared as a tea.

Important Considerations The hairs on mullein have been noted to cause irritation to the mouth and throat. To avoid this potential discomfort, filter remedies containing mullein before taking them.

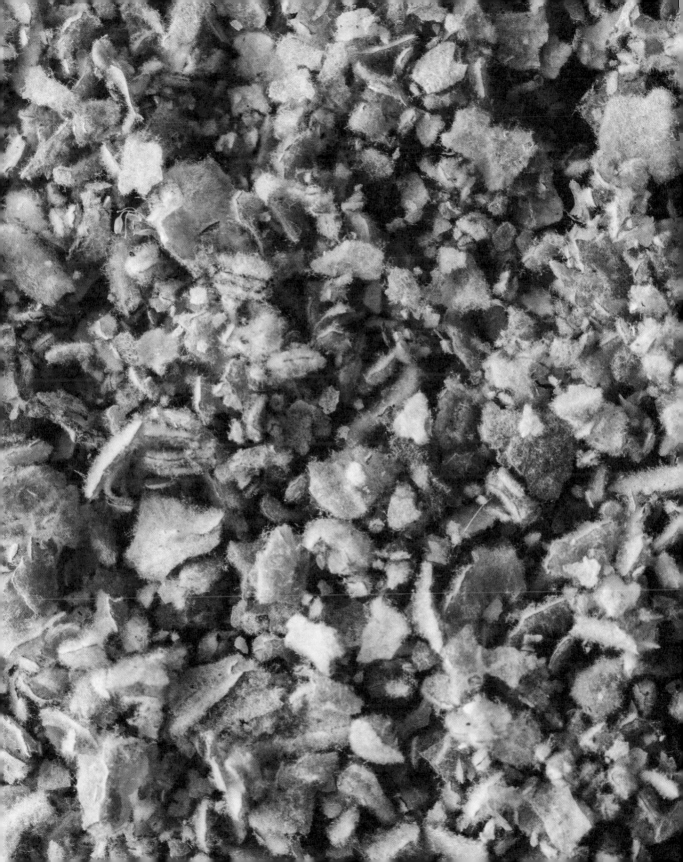

Nettle

Urtica dioica

The nettle plant is commonly called stinging nettle, and many people tend to avoid it in nature because of its painful bite. However, the sting from a stinging nettle can be used to ease arthritis inflammation and pain. Hitting oneself with nettle to achieve this effect is called urtication, which ties back to the plant's Latin name.

Why I Love This Herb Nettle might just be my all-time favorite herb to work with. I take medicinals I craft with nettles to ease my allergies; a long steep of nettles and oatstraw (with or without local honey, depending on the severity of my allergy symptoms) helps ease my suffering. Nettle is a powerful nervine and has helped me through a long recovery from massive adrenal fatigue and nervous system depletion.

Qualities Nettle is a diuretic, astringent (shrinks/tightens body tissues), anti-inflammatory, tonic (maintains the balance of systems over a long period of time), and prevents hemorrhage/bleeding.

Plant Family Urticaceae

Medicinal Parts Seeds, leaves, and roots (fresh and dried)

Ideal for Addressing As a nervine, nettle is most commonly used to help relieve allergy discomfort. It can also treat anemia, eczema, and arthritis pain including gout.

Most Common Preparations Nettle is most commonly prepared as a tea, but it frequently appears as decoctions and tinctures, in creams, and in certain food preparations.

Important Considerations Pregnant and nursing people as well as people taking blood pressure medication, should avoid taking nettle due to its diuretic properties.

Orange

Citrus sinensis

Although California and Florida are known for their bountiful production of oranges, it is believed that the sweet orange originated in China. Dried orange peel contributes to many formulations and single-ingredient remedies in both traditional Chinese medicine and Western herbalism.

Why I Love This Herb Much like dried lemon peel, dried orange peel offers a sweet aroma that brightens energy while also making the air feel fresher and cleaner. I like to mix dried orange peels and dried lemon peels together to create a summertime room steamer to clear stagnant air.

Qualities Dried orange peel is warming and drying. It is an aromatic and a bitter that stimulates appetite and aids digestion.

Plant Family Rutaceae

Medicinal Parts Peel

Ideal for Addressing Dried orange peels help boost the immune system. The flavonoids in the peels help maintain healthy blood pressure levels as well as healthy cholesterol levels.

Most Common Preparations Tinctures and glycerites are the most common preparations.

Important Considerations Do not take dried orange peel if you have a citrus allergy. It also may negatively interact with some antibiotics, chemotherapy drugs, and beta blockers. If you take any of these medications, speak to your healthcare provider about possible interactions.

Parsley

Petroselinum crispum

Parsley is native to Europe and the Eastern Mediterranean area. It grows prolifically around the globe in temperate climates. It was once a wild plant, but now it is rare to find it outside of commercial growing environments.

Why I Love This Herb I do not often work with parsley, opting for its spicier and more aromatic relative, cilantro. However, when I do, I love to add it to my medicinal pestos, my healing soup broths, and my fresh-pressed juices.

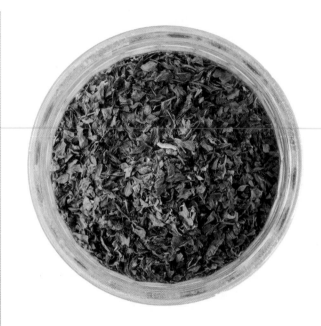

Qualities Parsley is antioxidative, a diuretic, and anti-inflammatory.

Plant Family Apiaceae

Medicinal Parts Leaves, roots, and seeds

Ideal for Addressing Parsley is a uterine stimulant and helps relieve menstrual cramps. It also helps balance digestion and ease trapped gas.

Most Common Preparations Parsley is often eaten fresh and as a culinary garnish, or as an addition to food preparation.

Important Considerations Excessive ingestion of parsley seeds can be toxic. Do not take parsley seeds if you are pregnant or if you have kidney problems.

Passionflower

Passiflora incarnata

The beautiful bloom of the passionflower looks like it fell out of the era of the dinosaurs. This flower has deep religious underpinnings; its orientation is thought to represent the crucifixion of Christ. Native to the Southern United States and to Central and South America, passionflower can be harvested all year long in warmer climates. It produces flowers even during its fruiting phase, so the flowers can be gathered fairly consistently. The fruits, called maypops, are edible when fully ripe and can be eaten fresh off the vine or made into jelly.

Why I Love This Herb I love the wild, spindly layers of the passionflower. Not only does it produce lovely fruit, but it also contributes to many types of herbal medicines.

Qualities Passionflower is a sedative, helps calm muscle spasms, and has tranquilizing properties.

Plant Family Passifloraceae

Medicinal Parts Flowers, leaves, and fruit

Ideal for Addressing Passionflower is noted for its gentle sedative properties.

Most Common Preparations Passionflower is most commonly crafted as a tea or a tincture.

Important Considerations Pregnant and nursing people should not take high doses of passionflower. Passionflower can cause drowsiness, so be careful when driving or doing activities that need full, sharp attention.

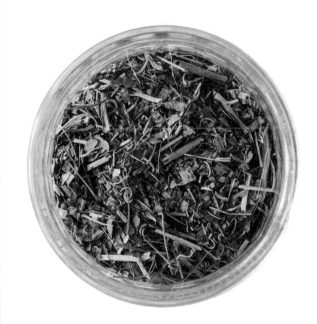

Peppermint

Mentha piperita L.

Peppermint is globally famous. What other medicinal herb has a candy named after it? A little-known fact about this well-known herb is that peppermint is actually a hybrid of spearmint and water mint. Though no one is truly sure where peppermint originated, dried peppermint leaves were found in an Egyptian pyramid dating back to around 1000 BCE.

Why I Love This Herb I love peppermint's cooling sensation. Whether as a tea, extract, or syrup, it is a flavor I enjoy. One of my favorite ways to take peppermint is in a simple cup of tea. Holding the warm mug between my hands and breathing in the refreshing aroma to open my airways is one of my life's little pleasures.

Qualities Peppermint is antimicrobial, analgesic, helps calm muscle spasms, and encourages sweating.

Plant Family Lamiaceae

Medicinal Parts Leaves

Ideal for Addressing Peppermint is especially good for ailments associated with the digestive system. It eases nausea, calms gas and bloating, relieves bowel spasms, and eases diarrhea.

Most Common Preparations Peppermint is most commonly prepared as a tea, though its essential oil is also widely used.

Important Considerations Peppermint is contraindicated for use in children under age 5, as it can cause breathing difficulties.

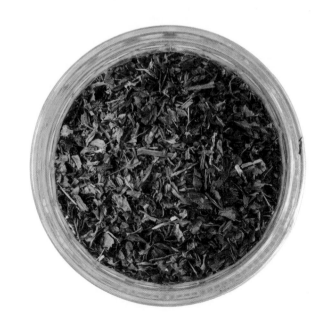

Pine

Pinus (genus name, as many types of pine can be used)

Pine needles come from the pine tree, which is coniferous and evergreen. Pine needles are long and slender (not flat) and grow in bundles of two, three, or five needles connected at their base. Pine needles can range in size from three to five inches. They have a strong pine scent and a sharp flavor. The pine most often included in teas and medicinals is the eastern white pine. Other types of pine in herbal medicine include Virginia pine, red pine, and sugar pine.

Why I Love This Herb I love pine needles for their sharp, green scent. I like to put them in a steamer on my stovetop. They have a lovely purifying effect on the air and make the entire space smell like a winter wonderland.

Qualities Pine is a decongestant, anti-inflammatory, antibacterial, antimicrobial, and anxiolytic (reduces anxiety).

Plant Family Pinaceae

Medicinal Parts Needles

Ideal for Addressing Pine needles are used to treat coughs, colds, phlegm, and sinus infections.

Most Common Preparations Pine needle tea is one of the most common preparations.

Important Considerations Pine needles are contraindicated in pregnancy. Be careful not to harvest yew or cypress needles, as they are not just toxic but also lethal when ingested. If you are unsure about a certain evergreen needle's toxicity, ask a professional or leave it alone.

Plantain

Plantago lanceolata and Plantago major

Plantain originates in Europe and the temperate zones of Asia. Originating in Europe and Asia, plantain was originally brought to North America as a valuable and revered medicinal herb and food source. The seeds of the plantain traveled swiftly, becoming such an accurate tool for noting where European colonizers had been that the plant became known as white man's footstep. Today, though many see it as a frustrating weed that perpetually invades their gardens and lawns, plantain is still revered by the herbal community as a very valuable plant.

Why I Love This Herb Plantain is a shockingly versatile one-plant first aid kit. My children know how to identify it, what it can be used for, and how to safely forage it to avoid pesticides, animal waste, and other yuck that is often found where plantain likes to grow.

Qualities Plantain is antibiotic, can help stop bleeding, and acts as a drawing agent ("draws" problems to the surface, such as splinters but also boils and pimples). It is also a diuretic, expectorant, and has antimucus properties.

Plant Family Plantaginaceae

Medicinal Parts Leaves

Ideal for Addressing Plantain can be used to cover a wound and stop bleeding. Chewing the plantain leaf and then placing it on the injured area creates a sort of field bandage. When ingested, plantain helps with gastritis, ulcers, irritable bowel syndrome, urinary tract infections, and even respiratory inflammation.

Most Common Preparations While plantain is sometimes engaged with in its unadulterated form, it is most often blended into tinctures and syrups.

Important Considerations Plantain contains high levels of vitamin K, which the body utilizes to aid in clotting. People who take blood thinners should consult their doctor before use.

Red Raspberry Leaf

Rubus idaeus

Red raspberry leaf is possibly one of the most well-known herbs for menstrual health and reproductive health. A member of the rose family, red raspberry leaf is indigenous to the temperate climates of Europe, Asia, and North America. It is packed with vitamins and minerals, including calcium, iron, magnesium, potassium, and zinc.

Why I Love This Herb I love this herb for its gentle strength and its lovely flavor. Red raspberry leaf tea is one of my favorite menstrual-time teas. It not only helps ease cramping and gastrointestinal discomfort, but it also seems to soothe the malaise I feel during that portion of my cycle.

Qualities Red raspberry leaf is astringent, antioxidative, and anti-inflammatory, contains anti-diarrhea properties, and has both stimulatory and relaxation effects on smooth muscle.

Plant Family Rosacea

Medicinal Parts Leaves

Ideal for Addressing Menstrual cramps, relaxing the uterus, balancing hormones, digestive support, oral health support (specifically mouth ulcers, sore throats, and gum disease), morning sickness, and labor pains

Most Common Preparations Teas and extracts

Important Considerations Red raspberry leaf should be avoided by people with hormone-sensitive conditions such as cancer, endometriosis, and uterine fibroids.

Skullcap

Scutellaria lateriflora

American skullcap (not to be confused with Baikal skullcap/Chinese skullcap) is indigenous to North America. It can be found in marshes, swamplands, and other wetland areas. A perennial mint, skullcap gets its name from the way in which its blue or violet flowers resemble tiny helmets. Skullcap was once thought to treat rabies and was known by the name "mad dog weed." Although it was found that skullcap does not cure rabies, it does help with anxiety and acts as a gentle relaxant.

Why I Love This Herb While skullcap is not my personal go-to nervine, I love how powerful, yet gentle, this herb can be. Skullcap is versatile and can assist with all types of nervous systems disorders, such as headaches, excessive stress, irritability, and a nervous mind.

Qualities Skullcap is diuretic, anti-inflammatory, antioxidant, antispasmodic (suppresses muscle spasms), and has sedative properties.

Plant Family Lamiaceae

Medicinal Parts Leaves and stems

Ideal for Addressing Skullcap can help with nerve tremors (such as those found with Parkinson's disease) and anxiety, and acts as a sedative.

Most Common Preparations Tea or tincture

Important Considerations Do not take if pregnant or nursing. Due to its sedative properties, skullcap should not be taken with medications that have similar properties, as this can cause excessively slow or difficult breathing or difficulty waking, and could lead to a need for medical attention. If you take any sedative medications, speak to your healthcare provider to check for any potential herb/drug interactions.

Turmeric

Curcuma longa

Turmeric, also known as curcumin, is a bright orange rhizome (a continuously growing horizontal underground stem) indigenous to India and Southeast Asia. A relative of ginger, turmeric is well known for its culinary, medicinal, and fabric-dyeing capabilities. It has been important to Ayurvedic healing practices for thousands of years.

Why I Love This Herb There isn't a day that goes by that I do not work with turmeric in my culinary and medicinal preparations. It has made its way into my cocoa, oatmeal, taco seasoning, teas, *everywhere*! I love its spicy aroma and its sharp, unique flavor. I craft a medicinal tea of ginger, turmeric, cinnamon, freshly ground black pepper, and honey whenever my gut becomes inflamed.

Qualities Turmeric is anti-inflammatory, antioxidant, helps regulate blood pressure, and has shown success in easing some forms of depression.

Plant Family Zingiberaceae

Medicinal Parts Rhizome (commonly known as the root)

Ideal for Addressing Turmeric assists in reducing inflammation, aids in digestion and relieving gas, and can help lower cholesterol.

Most Common Preparations Turmeric is most commonly prepared as a hot beverage such as golden milk or tea. Medicinally, it is most often taken in powder form mixed with other herbs or in capsules.

Important Considerations People with liver or bile duct disorders should not take turmeric, as it can increase bile production.

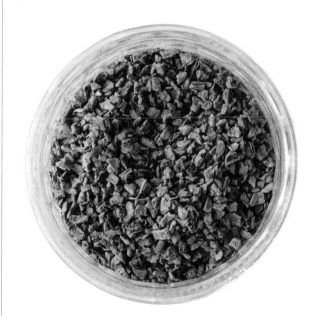

White Willow Bark

Salix alba

White willow bark is indigenous to Europe and Western Asia and has been naturalized in some parts of North America, Northern Asia, and much of Africa. White willow is a deciduous tree that loves water and thrives in wet conditions. The bark of the white willow tree was crafted into medicine by the Indigenous people of North America, who chewed it to soothe aches and pains. In 1828, Johann Andreas Buchner at the University of Munich isolated the active ingredient in white willow bark and named it salicin. In 1897, the research of German chemist Felix Hoffmann enabled the Bayer company to create the first pharmaceutically crafted aspirin in 1899. However, unlike its chemical mimicker, white willow bark works in a broader way in pain remediation and will not harm the gastrointestinal mucosa.

Why I Love This Herb White willow bark is amazing to me. Its herbal powers were so obvious that Western science and medicine created aspirin from its most active ingredient. Aspirin has been used to save lives (for people who suffer from heart attacks) and ease pain.

Qualities White willow bark is a pain reliever, anti-inflammatory, and fever reducer.

Plant Family Salicaceae

Medicinal Parts Bark

Ideal for Addressing Pain relief

Most Common Preparations Tea or tincture

Important Considerations Do not take white willow bark if you are allergic to aspirin or to medications with salicylate in them. Do not give to children or teens who could have a viral infection, as white willow bark can trigger Reye's syndrome (a rare reaction that can cause liver damage, confusion, and swelling of the brain). Do not take if pregnant or nursing.

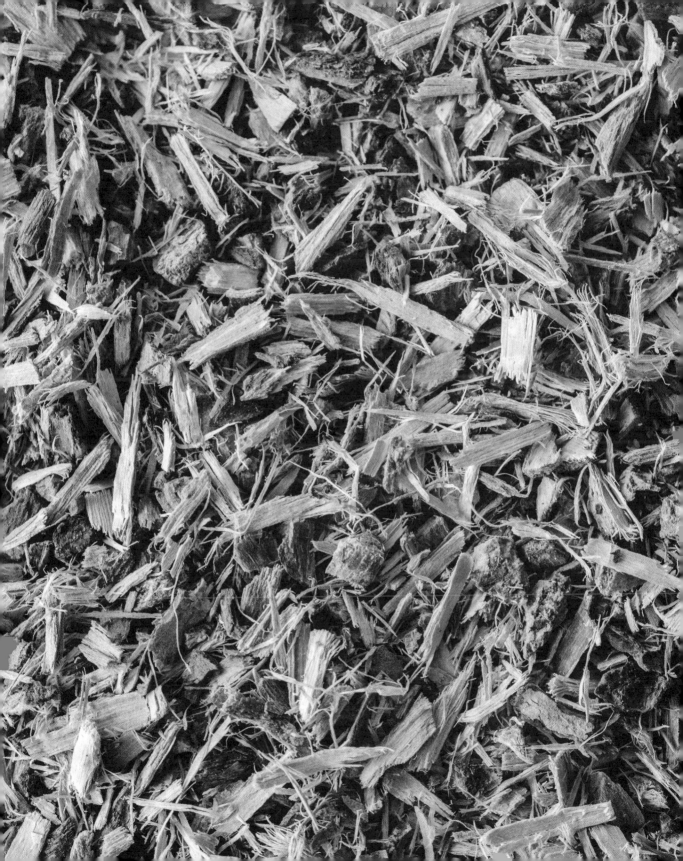

Yarrow

Achillea millefolium

Another relative of the daisy, yarrow has clusters of tiny five-petaled flowers growing atop long stalks with thin, featherlike leaves. While yarrow flowers can come in a rainbow of colors, in nature they are most often white or pale yellow. This lovely medicinal has several look-alikes, one of which is dangerous and potentially deadly: poison hemlock. Poison hemlock can cause major illness and death if ingested. Be aware, and beware if foraging! When in doubt, don't pick, don't ingest.

Why I Love This Herb I am deeply impressed by yarrow's ability to heal on very different levels. Yarrow on the skin can help heal wounds, and yarrow, when ingested, helps with inflammation. It also works on the nervous system, easing anxiety, and as a sedative to alleviate insomnia.

Qualities Yarrow is anti-inflammatory, has sedative and antimicrobial properties, and helps stop bleeding.

Plant Family Asteraceae

Medicinal Parts Flowers and leaves

Ideal for Addressing Yarrow works to stop the bleeding of cuts and wounds, increases the production of saliva and stomach acid to improve digestion, and can be crafted into body products to aid in skin health.

Most Common Preparations Teas and tinctures

Important Considerations Do not take if pregnant or nursing.

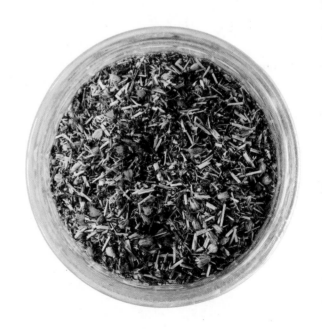

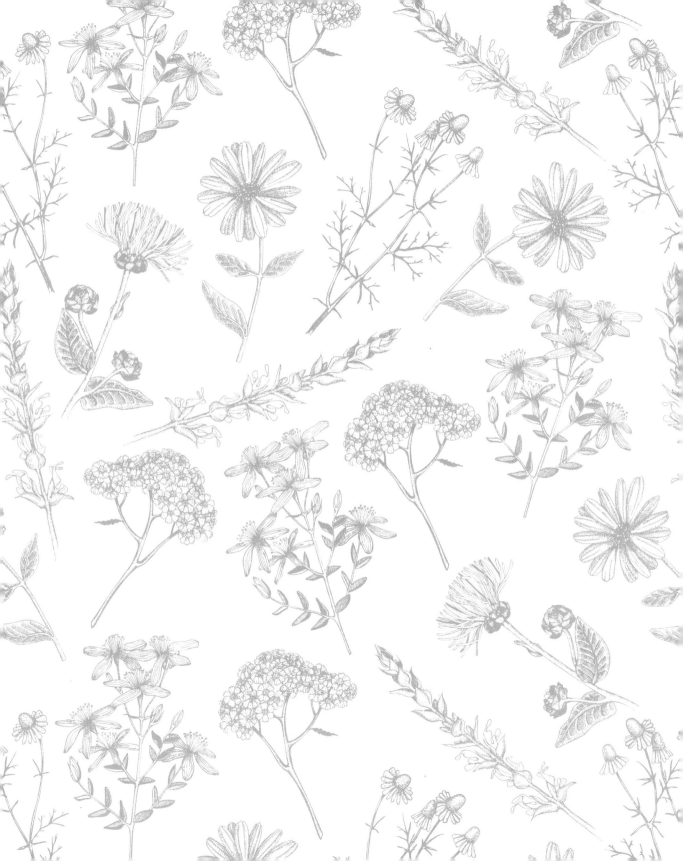

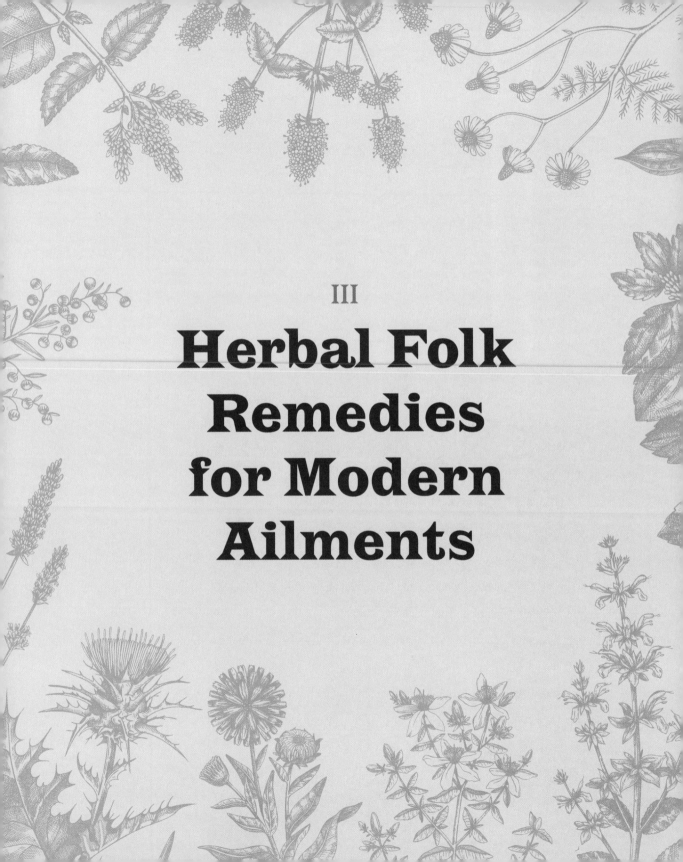

III

Herbal Folk Remedies for Modern Ailments

Hello, my loves—you have made it! Here we will discuss the modern-day stressors that can impinge upon your health and explore remedies you can craft to restore yourself to a more balanced state. This part of the book is organized so you can scan through different sections to see which remedies might best suit your particular needs. Each section speaks to the various ways in which your health can be disrupted, be it through environmental toxicity or inborn maladies. You can also scan through the table of contents at the front of the book, where you may find other remedies and symptoms similar to the condition you are treating. May this section help you create the wellness you seek.

Protecting against Environmental and Lifestyle Stressors

Especially in modern times, each of us is exposed to many external health influences beyond our control—things like air pollution, environmental toxins (such as fertilizers and other poisons in our water systems), household molds, fungus, and dust particulates from the breakdown of the home. Likewise, we are exposed to lifestyle stressors. Some of these stressors we can control, such as sitting overly long, standing without movement (which is equally harmful), lack of sleep, and stressful work, social, and home environments. In this section, I dig into a few common environmental and lifestyle stressors and share remedies and herbal allies that can be used to protect against them.

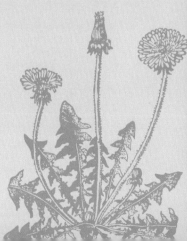

DANDELION

UNHEALTHY AIR QUALITY

Unhealthy air quality is a constant environmental exposure concern for each of us. Be it from the smog pollution from factories in urban environments and the farming industry in rural areas, to smoke and ash from yearly wildfires (which are becoming more and more frequent due to the extreme drought and heat conditions brought about by the climate crisis), to emissions from our vehicles and the fuels burned to run our daily lives, and even to indoor air pollutants like chemically scented candles and cleaning products, there are a multitude of ways in which our lungs are being exposed to potential harm and damage.

Here are some symptoms associated with exposure to unhealthy air quality:

- Burning, dry, painful eyes
- Coughing and wheezing
- Increased risk of cardiovascular disease
- Increased upper-respiratory infections
- New and/or increased asthma attacks
- Pain, burning, or discomfort in the chest, especially when attempting to take a deep breath
- Tight, shallow breathing
- Sore, burning throat, with difficulty swallowing

There are some wonderful herbal remedies you can craft to protect against the harms of exposure to unhealthy air quality.

Respiratory Steam for Inhalation
YIELDS 3 CUPS HERB MIX (FOR 3 TO 6 STEAMS)

Inhaled herbal steams allow the body to take in a remedy directly where it is needed, at the time it is needed. Respiratory steams are great for congestion caused by illness as well as for aggravated breathing due to environmental impact such as from fires.

INGREDIENTS*
½ **cup chamomile flower**
½ **cup eucalyptus leaf**
½ **cup lavender flower**
½ **cup peppermint leaf**
½ **cup pine needles**
½ **cup thyme leaf**

Ingredients are dried unless otherwise indicated.

INSTRUCTIONS
1. In a medium bowl, stir together all the herbs until mixed thoroughly. Transfer to a 32-ounce glass mason jar and seal the jar with a tight-fitting lid. Label and date the jar.

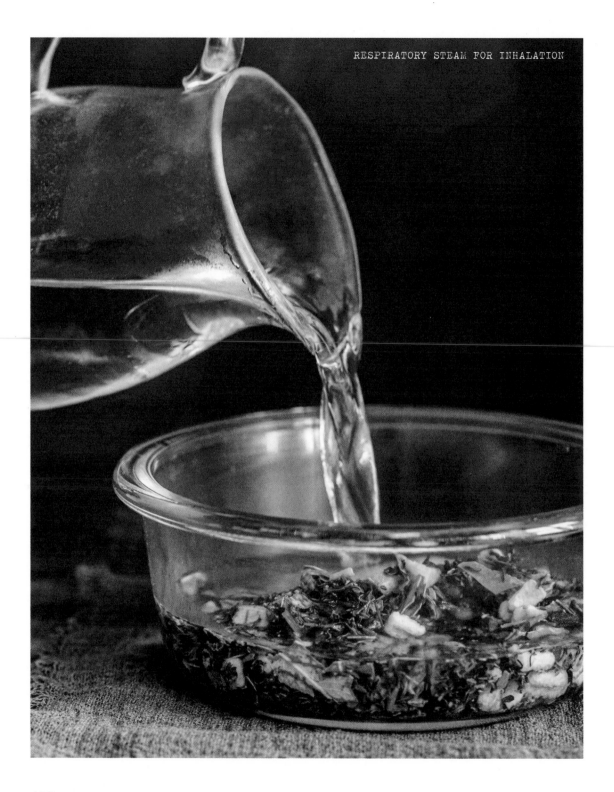

HERBAL MEDICINE FOR MODERN LIFE

2. To prepare a steam, in a medium pot, bring 4 to 6 cups of water to a boil over high heat. Scoop ½ to 1 cup of herb mix into the boiling water. Turn off the heat and stir the water gently until the herbs are submerged. Cover and let steep for 20 to 30 minutes.

3. When the remedy is ready, grab two towels. Lay one folded towel on a sturdy, heatproof surface and carefully place the pot on it. Drape the remaining towel over your head and the pot, covering any gaping openings so the steam stays trapped under the towel with you. Lean 5 to 10 inches away from the pot, being careful not to burn yourself, close your eyes, breathe deeply, and let the steam soothe your lungs, sinuses, eyes, and skin. Steam for at least 5 to 10 minutes, but no more than 15 minutes in one sitting.

SUGGESTED USE/DOSAGE

Steam for as long as you are able, but no longer than 15 minutes at a time. Steam as needed, but not more than once an hour, so the herbs do their work while giving the body time to relax between treatments.

WARNING *Do not use pine needles if you are pregnant. Do not use with children under 5 years of age.*

Lung Support Tea

YIELDS ABOUT 10 TABLESPOONS HERB MIX (FOR 10 CUPS OF TEA)

This tea is filled with gentle yet powerful herbal allies that support lung function and ease breathing aggravation. The herbs in this tea act as expectorants, dry out mucus, and are good for opening the airways.

INGREDIENTS*

3 tablespoons elecampane root
2 tablespoons mullein leaf
2 tablespoons marshmallow root
1 tablespoon peppermint leaf
1 tablespoon chamomile flower
1½ teaspoons fenugreek seed
1½ teaspoons ginger root
½ teaspoon thyme leaf

Ingredients are dried unless otherwise indicated.

INSTRUCTIONS

1. In a small bowl, stir together all the herbs until mixed thoroughly. Transfer to a 16-ounce glass mason jar and seal the jar with a tight-fitting lid. Label and date the jar.

2. To prepare the tea, place 1 tablespoon herb mix into a tea strainer or loose-leaf tea bag and into a mug (or place the mix directly in the mug). Pour 1 cup just-boiled water over the herbs and let steep for

30 minutes to 1 hour. This will give you a very strong herbal tea. (The longer you steep the herbs, the more oils that are extracted and present in your remedy.)

3. Strain through a fine-mesh strainer lined with cheesecloth. Drink and enjoy.

SUGGESTED USE/DOSAGE
Drink 2 to 3 cups a day for up to 3 weeks. Take 1 week to rest before continuing as needed or desired.

WARNING *If you take any medications, talk to your healthcare provider before using this remedy. Marshmallow root can disrupt the ability of medications to be absorbed and has also shown blood sugar–lowering properties, so do not use if you take diabetes medication. Ginger should not be taken by people who have a bleeding disorder or are taking blood thinners. Do not give to children under 5 years of age. Be mindful if you are allergic to plants in the Asteraceae and/or Compositae families as elecampane and chamomile could trigger an allergic reaction. Large doses of elecampane can cause nausea, vomiting, diarrhea, and abdominal cramping. Fenugreek is contraindicated for pregnancy.*

Lung Support Oxymel

YIELDS ABOUT 8 FLUID OUNCES (48 DOSES)

An oxymel is a vinegar-and-honey herbal blend, a deliciously sweet way to ingest herbal remedies. This oxymel is made up of herbs that are antispasmodics (help calm muscle spasms), expectorants, useful for drying mucus in the lungs, and good for opening the airways.

INGREDIENTS*
½ **teaspoon wild cherry bark**
½ **teaspoon mullein leaf**
½ **teaspoon peppermint leaf**
½ **teaspoon rose petals**
½ **teaspoon elecampane root**
½ **cup raw apple cider vinegar**
½ **cup raw honey (local and organic if possible)**

Ingredients are dried unless otherwise indicated.

INSTRUCTIONS

1. In a 16-ounce glass mason jar, combine all the herbs. Pour in the vinegar and honey and seal the jar with a tight-fitting lid (if using a metal lid, put a piece of parchment paper between the jar and lid so the vinegar doesn't corrode the metal). Shake the mixture thoroughly. Put the jar in a cool, dark, dry place

for about 2 weeks, shaking it every 2 to 3 days.

2. Strain the oxymel into an 8-ounce glass mason jar and seal the jar with a tight-fitting lid. Label and date the jar. A properly sealed oxymel is shelf stable for 1 year, unopened. Once opened, it will last up to 6 months so long as it is not contaminated.

SUGGESTED USE/DOSAGE

Take 1 teaspoon (5 mL) 2 to 3 times a day. For more acute symptoms, take 3 dropperfuls (3 mL) 5 times a day.

WARNING *Do not give to children under 5 years of age. Be mindful if you are allergic to plants in the Asteraceae and/or Compositae families as elecampane could trigger an allergic reaction.*

Soothing Herbal Eye Wash

YIELDS 1⅓ CUPS HERB MIX (FOR 64 EYE WASHES)

Eyewashes are used to assist with many eye wellness needs. This eyewash soothes irritation, inflammation, dryness, itchiness, and discomfort brought about by the eye's contact with foreign objects, such as bugs, dirt, dust, and smoke.

INGREDIENTS*

⅓ **cup marshmallow root**
⅓ **cup plantain leaf**
⅓ **cup calendula flower**
⅓ **cup red raspberry leaf**

Ingredients are dried unless otherwise indicated.

INSTRUCTIONS

1. In a medium bowl, stir together all the herbs until mixed thoroughly. At this point, you can either make individual tea bags or place the herb mixture into a 16-ounce glass mason jar until needed and seal the jar with a tight-fitting lid.

2. To make individual tea bags, you will need 64 heat-sealable tea bags. Fill each bag with 1 teaspoon of herb mix. Heat an iron on the cotton setting. Iron the open end of the bag to seal it, being careful not to iron over the herbs inside. Check that the seal is closed. Store the bags in an airtight container.

3. To prepare the eyewash, place 1 teaspoon of herb mix (or 1 tea bag) into a heatproof container. Pour 1 cup just-boiled water over the herbs, cover, and steep for 15 minutes.

4. Strain the remedy (or remove the tea bag) into a sanitized container

and let the rinse cool to room temperature so it does not injure your eyes or face.

5. Wash your eyes with the wash. (If using your hand as the container, place your open eye into the liquid, blink several times, then try to keep your eye open in the eyewash for 1 minute.)

SUGGESTED USE/DOSAGE
Wash your eyes once a day, as needed, and up to 3 times a day for more chronic symptoms.

WARNING *Avoid red raspberry leaf if you have any hormone-sensitive conditions, such as cancer, endometriosis, or uterine fibroids.*

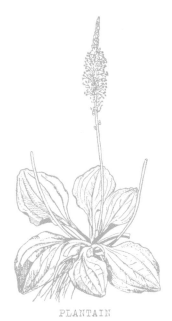

PLANTAIN

EXCESSIVE SITTING AND STANDING

These days, many of us live a life of extremes. Many people work long hours at multiple jobs that require prolonged periods of sitting or static standing (standing with no energetic movement). While many of us are aware of how harmful long periods of sitting can be, I doubt many people know that excessive standing can be equally harmful.

According to medical studies, more than an hour of sustained sitting is harmful to the body in a multitude of ways. Excessive sitting on a regular basis can lead to these issues:

- Back, neck, and hip pain
- Deep vein thrombosis
- Diabetes
- Edema
- High blood pressure
- Increased anxiety
- Varicose veins

Excessive standing, defined as more than four hours of inactive standing (experienced by door greeters, security workers, cashiers, etc.) can lead to multiple health hazards, including:

- Cardiac disorders
- Carotid arteriosclerosis
- Collapsed arches

- Dizziness
- Edema of the lower extremities
- Extreme fatigue
- Foot and ankle problems
- Increased risk of preterm birth (for pregnant people)
- Lower back pain
- Low blood pressure
- Orthostatic intolerance
- Varicose veins

Stretching, resting, and changing positions regularly can help keep your body feeling good and diminish the effects of these inactivity issues. Unfortunately, it is not always possible to take care of oneself in a work setting, especially if you drive a bus, stand at a register for eight-hour shifts, or work any number of service industry jobs. Herbal remedies can assist in staving off harmful effects and keeping your body happy and healthy.

High Blood Pressure Broth

YIELDS ABOUT 5 CUPS

Nothing warms the body and soothes the soul quite like a cup of broth. Overflowing with garlic goodness, this broth is filled with allicin. As the main compound in garlic, allicin helps lower blood pressure by preventing the body's production of the hormone angiotensin, which contracts the blood vessels. In bringing garlic together with the anti-inflammatory properties of turmeric and the chemical properties in celery that help relax artery walls and increase healthy blood flow, this broth will not only warm your heart but also aid in your BP health! Sip as is or add cooked noodles, rice, an egg, or vegetables to the broth.

INGREDIENTS

1 tablespoon extra-virgin olive oil
20 garlic cloves, smashed
¼ cup chopped celery
½ yellow onion
1 (2- to 3-inch) piece fresh ginger, peeled and grated
2 teaspoons dried parsley flakes, or 2 tablespoons fresh parsley leaf
2 teaspoons dried thyme leaf, or 2 tablespoons fresh thyme
1 teaspoon turmeric powder
¼ teaspoon freshly ground black pepper (omit if allergic)
Sea salt

INSTRUCTIONS

1. In a large soup pot with a lid over medium heat, heat the olive oil. Add the garlic and fry lightly for 2 to 3 minutes. You do not want it to brown. Add the celery, onion,

ginger, parsley, thyme, turmeric, and pepper and cook, stirring occasionally, for another minute.

2. Add 5 cups water and 1 teaspoon of salt. Cover the pot and let simmer for 20 minutes.

3. Strain the broth through a fine-mesh strainer into a heatproof bowl, pressing the solids against the strainer to get out all the liquid. Taste and season to taste with salt. Refrigerate in an airtight container for up to 4 days.

SUGGESTED USE/DOSAGE

Several times a day, warm 1 cup of broth, as warm as you can stand it, and sip. Incorporate the broth, or other garlic-heavy items, into your diet over multiple days throughout the week to increase your blood pressure stability and health.

WARNING *Ginger should not be taken by people who have a bleeding disorder or are taking blood thinners.*

Low Blood Pressure Tea

YIELDS 1 CUP HERB MIX (FOR 16 CUPS OF TEA)

Licorice root has long been known as an herb that increases blood pressure, so it is the perfect herb to provide a lovely remedy for people dealing with low blood pressure. Licorice root combined with tulsi (also known as holy basil) and cinnamon (known for its blood pressure–balancing properties) results in an aromatic and delicious beverage that will help bring your low blood pressure into balance.

INGREDIENTS*
½ **cup tulsi leaf**
¼ **cup licorice root**
¼ **cup cinnamon chips**

Ingredients are dried unless otherwise indicated.

INSTRUCTIONS

1. In a small bowl, stir together the tulsi leaf, licorice root, and cinnamon chips. Transfer to an 8-ounce glass mason jar and seal the jar with a tight-fitting lid. Label and date the jar.

2. To prepare the tea, place 1 tablespoon herb mix into a tea strainer or loose-leaf tea bag and into a mug (or place the mix directly in the mug). Pour 1 cup just-boiled water over the herbs and let steep for 5 minutes—longer if you want a stronger cup but no more than 10 minutes.

3. Strain as needed and enjoy.

For best results, drink the tea in the morning before eating.

WARNING *If you take blood pressure medications, consult your healthcare provider before using this remedy to avoid potential herb/drug contraindications. Limit cinnamon use during pregnancy.*

Dandelion Chai Latte for Edema

YIELDS ABOUT 1¼ CUPS HERB MIX (FOR 20 CUPS OF LATTE)

Dandelion root is a powerfully nourishing medicinal plant. It is a strong system detoxifier, filled with vitamins and minerals, and has diuretic, anti-inflammatory, and antioxidant properties. This tea is a delicious way to encourage your body to release excess fluids naturally that can gather due to prolonged sitting and standing.

INGREDIENTS*
1 cup dandelion root
16 cardamom pods
¼ cup ginger root
5 whole star anise
2 teaspoons vanilla bean powder (optional)
Honey or other natural sweetener, for sweetening (optional)
Dairy or nondairy beverage (I love my handcrafted oat milk for this as it is creamy and semisweet on its own), for serving (optional)

Ingredients are dried unless otherwise indicated.

INSTRUCTIONS

1. In a dry skillet over medium-high heat, roast the dandelion root, stirring frequently, until it turns a darker shade of brown and has a lovely aromatic smell. Let cool completely before transferring to a 16-ounce sanitized glass mason jar, so the heat does not create steam and ruin your herbal mix with condensation.

2. In a clean coffee grinder or using a mortar and pestle, grind the cardamom pods and add them to the cooled dandelion root. Add the ginger, star anise, and vanilla (if using) and seal the jar with a tight-fitting lid. Label and date the jar.

3. To prepare the latte, in a medium saucepan over medium heat, combine ¼ cup herb mix (making sure to grab only 1 star anise) and 4 cups water. Bring to a boil and boil for 5 to 6 minutes. Strain into a 32-ounce glass mason jar. Add honey

(if using) and milk (if using) to taste to create a medicinal latte.

SUGGESTED USE/DOSAGE

Drink as needed, up to 3 cups a day.

WARNING *Cardamom is contraindicated, in large doses, for pregnant people and people taking blood thinners. Ginger should not be taken by people who have a bleeding disorder or are taking blood thinners.*

Blood Sugar–Balancing Tincture

YIELDS ABOUT 10 FLUID OUNCES (150 TO 300 DOSES)

With the anti-inflammatory properties of turmeric, the blood sugar–lowering and –balancing properties of sencha (and all) green tea, and both fenugreek and cinnamon's insulin-sensitizing effects, this tincture is packed full of herbs that work to keep blood sugar in balance.

INGREDIENTS*

2 tablespoons fenugreek powder

2 tablespoons turmeric powder

2 tablespoons green sencha tea leaf

1 tablespoon cinnamon powder

½ teaspoon freshly ground black pepper (omit if allergic)

1¼ cups 80-proof vodka

Ingredients are dried unless otherwise indicated.

INSTRUCTIONS

1. In a 16-ounce glass mason jar, combine all the herbs. Pour in the vodka, seal the jar with a tight-fitting lid, and shake gently. Place the jar in a cool, dark, dry place for 6 to 8 weeks, shaking it 3 to 4 times a week.

2. Strain the tincture through a fine-mesh strainer lined with cheesecloth and set over a bowl and use a funnel to transfer it into one amber glass dropper bottle and amber glass tincture bottles with twist caps. Label and date the bottles.

SUGGESTED USE/DOSAGE

Take 1 to 2 dropperfuls (1 to 2 mL) 1 to 3 times a day as needed, or add to 1 cup cold or room-temperature water. Pay attention to how your body responds and adjust your intake accordingly.

WARNING *If you take blood pressure medications, consult your healthcare provider before using this remedy to avoid potential herb/drug contraindications. Avoid this remedy (cinnamon and fenugreek) during pregnancy. Avoid (green tea) if you take MAOIs (monoamine oxidase inhibitors).*

Warming Pain-Relief Balm

YIELDS 6 OUNCES

This soothing balm is great for soothing aches and pains from overuse or minor injury. The anti-inflammatory properties of turmeric and the warming properties of cayenne are wrapped up in soothing, healing coconut oil and cacao butter to create a winning and wonderful healing rub. I suggest wearing food-safe disposable gloves when crafting the balm. Turmeric will stain your hands a lovely shade of yellow-orange and cayenne could cause uncomfortable heat on your skin.

INGREDIENTS

- ½ **cup plus 2 tablespoons extra-virgin coconut oil**
- 2 **teaspoons turmeric powder**
- 2 **teaspoons cayenne pepper**
- ⅛ **teaspoon freshly ground black pepper**
- 2 **tablespoons beeswax pellets**
- 1½ **teaspoons cocoa butter**

INSTRUCTIONS

1. In a double boiler over low heat, combine the coconut oil, turmeric, cayenne, and black pepper. Heat for 1 hour to infuse the oil.

2. Place a fine-mesh strainer over a heatproof bowl and line the strainer with cheesecloth. Pour the warm infusion into the cheesecloth, letting the oil strain through. Squeeze the cheesecloth over the strainer to extract all the oil infusion.

3. Add the beeswax pellets and cacao butter to the strained oil infusion and place the bowl over the double boiler over low heat. Warm, stirring and watching constantly, until the mixture is melted and combined. Do not let it boil. Immediately pour the melted oil into two 3-ounce glass mason jars. Let sit, untouched, for 3 to 4 hours, or until the oils have set and solidified. Seal the jars with tight-fitting lids. Label and date the jars.

SUGGESTED USE/DOSAGE

If this is your first time using this, rub a small amount of the balm on the inside of your arm and wait 24 hours to check for potential reactions. To use, rub a small amount of the balm onto the affected area, massaging it into your skin thoroughly. Apply as needed, up to 4 times a day per area.

WARNING *Avoid any open cuts, rashes, burns, or soft tissue/mucous tissue zones, such as genitals, eyes, and the inside of your nose.*

DIGITAL FATIGUE

Digital fatigue is another lifestyle stressor that has become commonplace for people of all ages. Here are some symptoms associated with digital fatigue and excessive screen exposure:

- Eye strain
- Headaches
- Muscle pain
- Sleep disruption

Creating healthier digital habits and adding herbal remedies that can support and strengthen the ocular system, ease muscle pain, and aid in balanced circadian rhythms will help ease the negative impact of digital excess.

Dreamland Tea

YIELDS 2½ CUPS HERB MIX (FOR 40 CUPS OF TEA)

Sleep disruption is a common symptom of screen overuse. This tea, made with gentle, soothing nervines, will help your system relax and regulate itself, which will help induce slumber and assist in maintaining a more balanced circadian rhythm.

INGREDIENTS*

½ **cup lavender flower**

½ **cup lemon balm leaf**

½ **cup hops flower**

½ **cup German chamomile flower**

½ **cup nettles leaf**

Lemon, for serving (optional)

Honey, for serving (optional)

Dairy or nondairy beverage, for serving (optional)

Ingredients are dried unless otherwise indicated.

INSTRUCTIONS

1. In a medium bowl, stir together all the herbs until mixed thoroughly. Transfer to a 32-ounce glass mason jar and seal the jar with a tight-fitting lid. Label and date the jar.

2. To prepare the tea, place 1 tablespoon herb mix into a tea strainer or loose-leaf tea bag and into a mug (or place the mix directly in the mug). Pour 1 cup just-boiled water over the tea and let steep for 3 to 5 minutes. Strain as needed.

3. Add lemon (if using), honey (if using), or dairy/nondairy beverage of choice (if using).

Fun sidenote: These herbs also make a lovely sparkling beverage! Steep the tea blend as directed and strain as needed. Cover and let cool. Combine 1 part tea with 2 parts unflavored sparkling water. Add sweetener, lemon, or a mint sprig as desired. Enjoy your nighttime mocktail and sweet dreams!

SUGGESTED USE/DOSAGE

Drink 1 cup a day, 1 hour before bedtime as needed.

WARNING *Avoid lemon balm if you have a sensitive thyroid or hypothyroidism. Avoid nettles leaf if you are pregnant, nursing, or taking blood pressure medication. Be mindful if you are allergic to plants in the Asteraceae and/or Compositae families as chamomile could trigger an allergic reaction.*

Bright Happy Eyes Tea

YIELDS 1½ CUPS HERB MIX (FOR 24 CUPS OF TEA)

Staring too long at a screen, a great novel, or a term paper can fatigue your eye muscles, creating pain and discomfort. Ease the strain with these herbal allies that work to nourish eye health, prevent macular degeneration, relax the blood vessels in the eyes, boost energy, and protect against oxidative stress.

INGREDIENTS*

½ **cup green tea leaves**

½ **cup fennel seed**

¼ **cup orange peel**

¼ **cup passionflower leaf**

Ingredients are dried unless otherwise indicated.

INSTRUCTIONS

1. In a medium bowl, stir together all the herbs until mixed thoroughly. Transfer to a 16-ounce glass mason jar and seal the jar with a tight-fitting lid. Label and date the jar.

2. To prepare the tea, place 1 tablespoon herb mix into a tea strainer or loose-leaf tea bag and into a mug (or place the mix directly in the mug). Pour 1 cup just-boiled water over the tea and let steep for 4 to 6 minutes. Strain as needed and enjoy.

SUGGESTED USE/DOSAGE

Drink 1 cup a day as needed.

WARNING *Avoid green tea if you take MAOIs (monoamine oxidase inhibitors). Pregnant and nursing people should not take high doses of passionflower.*

Aches and Pains Rub

YIELDS 6 OUNCES

When you are dealing with physical aches and pains, this rub—filled with herbs that have analgesic, anti-inflammatory, and skin-healing properties—will help soothe them.

INGREDIENTS*

½ **cup plus 2 tablespoons extra-virgin olive oil**

2 **tablespoons arnica flower**

1 **tablespoon cayenne pepper**

1 **tablespoon comfrey leaf**

1 **tablespoon plantain leaf**

1 **tablespoon lavender flower**

1 **tablespoon calendula flower**

2 **tablespoons beeswax pellets**

2 **tablespoons cocoa butter**

2 **tablespoons unrefined shea butter**

Ingredients are dried unless otherwise indicated.

INSTRUCTIONS

1. In a double boiler over low heat, combine the olive oil, arnica, cayenne, comfrey, plantain, lavender, and calendula. Heat for 1 hour to infuse the oil.

2. Place a fine-mesh strainer over a heatproof bowl and line the strainer with cheesecloth. Pour the infused oil into the cheesecloth, letting the oil strain through. Squeeze the cheesecloth over the strainer to extract all the oil.

3. Add the beeswax pellets, cacao butter, shea butter to the strained oil and place the bowl over the double boiler over low heat. Warm, stirring and watching constantly, until the mixture is melted and combined. Do not let it boil. Immediately pour the melted oil into two 3-ounce glass mason jars. Let sit, untouched, for 3 to 4 hours, or until the oils have set and solidified. Seal the jars with tight-fitting lids. Label the jars.

SUGGESTED USE/DOSAGE

Rub the balm onto affected areas as often as needed.

WARNING *Do not apply to broken skin. Topical applications containing calendula are considered safe during pregnancy and while nursing but avoid the chest area so nurslings do not unintentionally ingest any salve. Arnica can cause contact dermatitis for people who have skin sensitivities and could trigger an allergic reaction if you are allergic to plants in the Asteraceae and/or Compositae families.*

ENVIRONMENTAL TOXIN EXPOSURE

As technology and agricultural businesses move ever forward, the by-products of those industries have begun to have harmful effects on the environment and on people. One of the most noticeable ways we are affected is by the increased presence of toxins and heavy metals in our bodies. These materials settle into our tissues and make it difficult for our bodies to detoxify themselves as well as cause our systems to function at less-than-optimal levels. Ingesting herbs that bind themselves to the toxins helps the body purge them more effectively so we can, once again, function at optimal health and wellness levels.

Symptoms of environmental toxin exposure vary from person to person, depending on what types of toxins a person is exposed to and for how long. Common symptoms associated with environmental toxin exposure include:

- Body aches
- Breathing complaints, including but not limited to
- coughing
- shortness of breath
- wheezing
- Contact dermatitis
- Headache
- Inflammation
- Major illness and even hospitalization associated with long-term exposure and/or systemic sensitivity
- Nausea
- Neurologic disorders

Heavy metal poisoning is serious, so if you are experiencing the symptoms listed or additional symptoms such as diarrhea, numbness or prickly sensations in the hands and feet, chills, low body temperature, abdominal pain, and feeling weak, seek medical care right away.

Heavy Metals Detox Tincture

YIELDS ABOUT 8 FLUID OUNCES (120 TO 240 DOSES)

Strengthen the systems that clear toxins from your body. Dandelion and red clover both boost liver function while also offering vitamins and minerals the body needs to maintain optimal health.

INGREDIENTS*
½ **cup red clover blossom**
½ **cup dandelion root**
1 **cup 80-proof vodka**

Ingredients are dried unless otherwise indicated.

INSTRUCTIONS

1. In a 16-ounce glass mason jar, combine the red clover and dandelion root. Pour in the vodka. Seal the jar with a tight-fitting lid and shake gently. Place the jar in a cool, dark, dry place for 6 to 8 weeks, shaking it 3 to 4 times a week.

2. Strain the tincture through a fine-mesh strainer set over a bowl and use a funnel to transfer it into amber glass tincture bottles. Label and date the bottles.

SUGGESTED USE/DOSAGE

Take 1 to 2 dropperfuls (1 to 2 mL) 3 to 4 times a day, or add to 1 cup water.

Heavy Metals Detox Soup

YIELDS 5 TO 6 CUPS

The dulse and cilantro in this soup bind to heavy metals, allowing the body to flush them. Dulse can also cross the blood-brain barrier, helping remove heavy metals from that area. Garlic contains sulfur, which helps the liver detoxify the entire system.

INGREDIENTS

1 tablespoon extra-virgin olive oil
4 to 6 garlic cloves, minced
4 small carrots, diced small
2 or 3 red radishes, diced small
1 bunch fresh green onions, sliced
1 bunch fresh cilantro, minced
⅓ cup dulse seaweed flakes (Atlantic red algae), minced
1 tablespoon dried mushrooms (maitake, shiitake, reishi, or a blend)
4½ cups water
Salt and freshly ground black pepper

INSTRUCTIONS

1. In a soup pot over medium heat, heat the olive oil. Add the garlic, carrots, radishes, green onions, and cilantro. Cook, stirring frequently, until the vegetables are tender, about 5 minutes.

2. Add the dulse and dried mushrooms and stir to combine well.

3. Add the water and bring to a boil. Reduce heat and simmer for 20 minutes. Season with salt and pepper.

4. Refrigerate leftovers in an airtight container for up to 4 days.

SUGGESTED USE/DOSAGE

The lovely thing about this soup is that you can eat it as often as you desire.

WARNING *Avoid dulse and other seaweed if you have hyperthyroidism, as high levels of iodine can be harmful.*

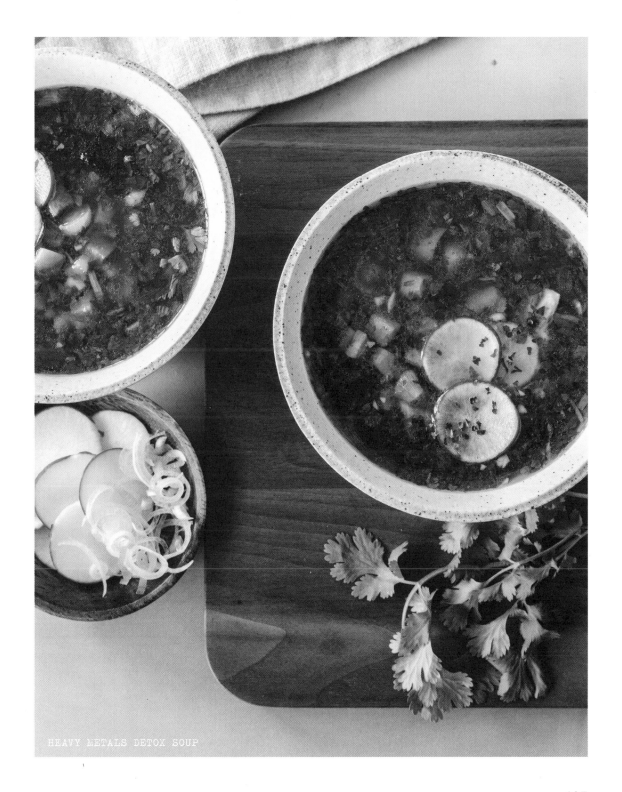

HEAVY METALS DETOX SOUP

Addressing Pharmaceutical and Dietary Effects

Pharmaceuticals have become a common part of our daily lives. Often, we use them without thinking, or in response to the constant onslaught of information from the media and our healthcare providers. I don't believe pharmaceutical medication is bad, but I think we need to have a more mindful relationship with it and how we use it.

Likewise, we are living in an era in which more processed food is available and ingested than at any other time in history. Finding balance and taking care of our bodies can be tricky, but it is imperative that we strike that balance for our health and well-being.

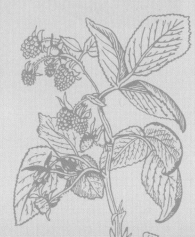

RASPBERRY

PRESCRIPTION AND ANTIBIOTIC SIDE EFFECTS

Western allopathic medicine, especially in recent years, has made great advances in the treatment of illness and disease. Unfortunately, the medications we take often have unpleasant, uncomfortable, and just plain irritating side effects. This is especially true when it comes to antibiotics, which move through the system killing good and bad bacteria indiscriminately. This can result in systemic candida overgrowth and diminished gut health. But take heart, it can be helped. One way to let your system heal is to take medications only as directed and when truly needed. You can also help get your system back into balance by adding herbal remedies that bolster gut health and healthy flora while staving off overgrowth of candida.

Gut Biome–Balancing Powder

YIELDS 3½ CUPS HERB POWDER (28 DOSES)

All sorts of medications can throw off the balance of your gut health. When your gut is out of whack, the imbalance can leave you feeling bloated, boggy, and like it is difficult to digest what you eat. The blend of gut-healing and nourishing herbs in this remedy will help ease the discomforts of leaky gut, gastritis, and other gut disruptions. Note, when purchasing fruit powder, make sure it is 100 percent fruit with no additives, preservatives, or sugars, as those ingredients can cause further gut distress.

INGREDIENTS

¾ **cup marshmallow root powder**

1½ **cups aloe vera leaf powder**

⅓ **cup cat's claw powder**

⅓ **cup meadowsweet powder**

¼ **cup green tea powder**

⅓ **cup fruit powder (I like blueberry or peach for their antioxidant properties and healthy fiber as well as their naturally sweet flavors)**

INSTRUCTIONS

In a medium bowl, stir together all the herb powders until mixed thoroughly. Transfer to a 32-ounce glass mason jar and seal the jar with a tight-fitting lid. Label and date the jar.

Mix 2 tablespoons powdered herb mix into your milk/nondairy beverage or a smoothie once a day.

WARNING *If you take any medications, talk to your healthcare provider before using this remedy. Marshmallow root can disrupt the ability of medications to be absorbed. Marshmallow has also shown blood sugar–lowering properties, so do not use if you take diabetes medication. Avoid green tea if you take MAOIs (monoamine oxidase inhibitors).*

Yeast-Be-Gone Capsules

YIELDS 345 CAPSULES (345 DOSES)

Candida overgrowth can create much discomfort and frustration in your life, in more ways than just thrush infections (vaginal yeast and oral yeast). Too much candida can cause brain fog, itchy and patchy skin, fatigue, and digestive issues. I recommend this herbal remedy, packed with astringent and antiviral herbs, to help clear your system.

INGREDIENTS*
¼ **cup pau d'arco powder**
¼ **cup black walnut hull powder**
¼ **cup clove powder**
¼ **cup ginger powder**
¼ **cup echinacea root powder**
3 **tablespoons red raspberry leaf, ground into a powder**
345 **empty size 00 capsules**

Ingredients are dried unless otherwise indicated.

INSTRUCTIONS

1. Cover your work surface with a towel.

2. In a medium bowl, stir together the herb powders until thoroughly blended. Transfer to a 16-ounce glass mason jar and label and date the jar. Reserve the bowl.

3. Transfer ¼ cup of the herb powder back into the bowl. Seal the larger jar with a tight-fitting lid.

4. Place a tray in the center of the work area and set the bowl of herb powder onto the tray. Gather the capsules and an 8-ounce glass mason jar for storing the filled capsules.

5. Working one at a time, open a capsule and use the long side of the capsule to scoop powder into the capsule, pushing it in and pressing it with your finger. When the capsule is full, place the other end of the capsule on and push it down to close. Rub a small amount of the herb remedy onto the outside of the

capsule before putting it into the jar. This allows your body to know what it is ingesting and prepare itself to digest and utilize the remedy. Seal the jar with a tight-fitting lid.

SUGGESTED USE/DOSAGE
Take 1 capsule a day for 7 to 10 days.

WARNING *Avoid red raspberry leaf if you have any hormone-sensitive conditions, such as cancer, endometriosis, or uterine fibroids. Echinacea is contraindicated for people who have an autoimmune disorder. Ginger should not be taken by people who have a bleeding disorder or are taking blood thinners. Also be mindful if you are allergic to plants in the Asteraceae and/ or Compositae families as it can trigger an allergic reaction.*

SELF-INDUCED SYSTEMIC OVERLOAD AND TOXICITY

These days, it seems like we're all living at a high level of intensity that is constantly skyrocketing. This motivates us to seek ways to bring ourselves back to calmer, more rational states of mind, often by self-medicating with sugar or alcoholic beverages. These habits become a quick and easy way to dull the noise and "buy some peace." I will not sit in judgment of anyone—I believe we all do the best we can with the tools we have. But, I will offer some herbal tools that can help when excess has gotten the best of you.

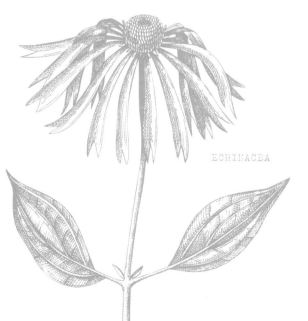

ECHINACEA

Hangover Ease and Liver Support Tincture

YIELDS 8 FLUID OUNCES (120 TO 240 DOSES)

The morning after exuberant drinking can feel like there is a conga line dancing through your brain while your gut decides how much of it wants to remain inside. No fun! The impact of alcohol on the body, especially on the liver, is fairly destructive—it kills liver cells and hampers the liver's ability to regenerate. This remedy, which includes herbs that stimulate the metabolism, can enhance detoxing. The herbs are also anti-inflammatory, ease digestive and bowel upset, and encourage healing and tissue regeneration.

INGREDIENTS*

¼ cup nettles leaf

3 tablespoons dandelion root

2 tablespoons ginger root

2 tablespoons fennel seed

2 tablespoons German chamomile flower

1 tablespoon peppermint leaf

1 tablespoon parsley leaf

1 tablespoon dried lemon peel

1 cup 80-proof vodka

Ingredients are dried unless otherwise indicated.

INSTRUCTIONS

1. In a 16-ounce glass mason jar, combine the herbs. Pour in the vodka, seal the jar with a tight-fitting led, and shake gently. Place the jar in a cool, dark, dry place for 6 to 8 weeks, shaking it several times a week.

2. Strain the tincture through a fine-mesh strainer set over a bowl and use a funnel to transfer it into one amber glass dropper bottle and amber glass tincture bottles with twist caps. Label and date the bottles.

SUGGESTED USE/DOSAGE

Take 1 to 2 dropperfuls (1 to 2 mL) a day, or add to 1 cup cold or room-temperature water, for 3 weeks, then take a week off. Pay attention to how your body responds to the remedy. Resume as needed.

WARNING *Use fennel with caution during pregnancy. Avoid nettles leaf if you are pregnant, nursing, or taking blood pressure medication. Ginger should not be taken if you have a bleeding disorder or take blood thinners. Do not give to children under 5 years of age. Be mindful if you are allergic to plants in the Asteraceae and/or Compositae families as chamomile could trigger an allergic reaction. Please note, this tincture is not a cure-all for struggles with* *alcohol. If you have a problem with alcohol, please seek help. Herbs can help the body heal up to a point, but consistent harm and damage from excessive drinking will take its toll. Be well, my friends!*

3-Ingredient Powder for Liver Support

YIELDS 1½ CUPS HERB POWDER (24 DOSES)

The three simple ingredients in this remedy are a knockout when combined. Working together, they have the remarkable properties of helping detoxify the liver, protecting against damage, assisting in regeneration, and improving liver function. I recommend wearing food-grade disposable gloves when crafting this remedy unless you want your hands to pick up the lovely green coloring of the powders.

INGREDIENTS

½ **cup wheatgrass powder**
½ **cup chlorella powder**
½ **cup spirulina powder**

INSTRUCTIONS

1. All of these herbal powders are light and airy and will waft away on the slightest breeze, so turn off fans and close windows in your workspace, and cover your work surface with a towel.

2. In a medium bowl, stir together the wheatgrass, chlorella, and spirulina powders gently until mixed thoroughly. Transfer to a 16-ounce glass mason jar and seal the jar with a tight-fitting lid. Label and date the jar.

SUGGESTED USE/DOSAGE

Stir 1 tablespoon herb powder into your smoothie, milk/nondairy beverage, or water a day as support after excess, and in general, to help the body detoxify.

Managing Physical Pain and Discomfort

Physical discomforts like pain, fatigue, and sleeplessness happen. And dealing with them can suck the energy out of you. Managing pain and discomfort with over-the-counter medications can relieve many symptoms, but they can also throw your system out of balance. This can be especially true for medications that lose their effectiveness if they are taken consistently over a long period of time, as the body builds up a tolerance to them. When this happens, people often start to increase the dose and experience some of the unpleasant side effects, which may include stomach pain and ulcers, increased blood pressure, nausea, dizziness, heartburn, and headaches. Luckily, there are herbs that can aid in symptom management while also nourishing the body.

ROSEMARY

144

FATIGUE

There is being tired, and then there is fatigue—exhaustion so strong it feels like you are being dragged down into deep water and are never quite able to break the surface. With so many things that can disrupt our rest and deplete our bodies and minds, fatigue is becoming a reality for more and more people. Taking time to nourish the systems that support you in feeling energized will help you beat fatigue and get your energy back.

Perk-Up Spray

YIELDS 4 FLUID OUNCES

When you need a little boost to perk you up, this spray will have you ready to go in a flash. Crafted from herbs known for reducing fatigue, lifting and brightening mood, increasing mental clarity, and stimulating the mind and body, a spritz or two will help put pep back in your step. Note that this is one of the more expensive recipes in this book, as essential oils tend to be pricey. But, I believe there is a "magic" to essential oils and scents—they have the power to change our states of mind quickly and effectively.

INGREDIENTS

1 tablespoon witch hazel

1 tablespoon vegetable glycerin

10 to 15 drops sweet orange essential oil

10 to 15 drops lemon essential oil

10 to 15 drops rosemary essential oil

10 to 15 drops basil essential oil

Distilled water, for filling the bottle

INSTRUCTIONS

1. Using a small funnel, pour the witch hazel and vegetable glycerin into a 4-ounce amber glass spray bottle.

2. Drop the essential oils into the liquid.

3. Fill the remaining space in the bottle with distilled water. Cap the bottle. Label and date it.

SUGGESTED USE/DOSAGE

Shake gently before use. Spray when you need a boost, avoiding the face.

Boost Me Herbal Mocha

YIELDS 6 TABLESPOONS HERB POWDER (FOR 6 CUPS OF MOCHA)

When you feel your energy flagging and you need to push through, this herbal mocha remedy will give you the boost you need without the nasty crash that can come from coffee or other energy-enhancement drinks or supplements. An added bonus is that the herbs in this drink have properties that help nourish your adrenals, boost your mood, and keep you feeling energized.

INGREDIENTS

¼ **cup raw cacao powder**

2 **teaspoons matcha powder**

2 **teaspoons maca powder**

1 **teaspoon vanilla powder (optional)**

1 **teaspoon cinnamon powder**

2 **tablespoons honey or honey granules (optional)**

INSTRUCTIONS

1. Gently sift each powder into an 8-ounce glass mason jar and stir gently to combine. Seal the jar with a tight-fitting lid. Label and date the jar.

2. To prepare the herbal mocha, in a small saucepan over medium heat, heat 1 cup milk/nondairy beverage, being careful it does not scorch. Remove from the heat.

3. Add 1 tablespoon herb powder and blend with an immersion blender until frothy. Alternatively, carefully pour the warm milk into a standard blend, add the powder, and blend. Pour into a mug and stir in the honey (if using). Sip and wake up joyfully!

SUGGESTED USE/DOSAGE

Drink as desired!

WARNING *If you take blood pressure medications, consult your healthcare provider before using this remedy to avoid potential herb/drug contraindications. Limit cinnamon use during pregnancy.*

FEVER AND CHILLS

Fevers are a natural part of the body's health defense system. On average, a fever can range anywhere from 99.5°F to 102°F before healthcare providers become concerned. I am a believer in letting a fever run its course. As a holistic wellness practitioner and mother of six (for twenty-six years now, as I write this), I have sat with my children and "nursed" them through many a fever without interfering. But there are certain moments, and certain fevers, that do make me nervous. It is in these times that I reach for remedies that help the body work through the fever while also helping fight off the germs causing it.

Fever-Ease Tea

YIELDS 1 CUP HERB MIX (FOR 24 TO 48 CUPS OF TEA)

This herbal remedy helps support healing by bringing down a fever, helping the body sweat, and easing the bowel upset occasionally associated with fever-related illness.

INGREDIENTS*

¼ **cup yarrow flower and leaf**

¼ **cup elderflower**

¼ **cup peppermint leaf**

2 **tablespoons fenugreek seed**

2 **tablespoons catnip**

Ingredients are dried unless otherwise indicated.

INSTRUCTIONS

1. In a small bowl, stir together all the herbs and seeds until mixed thoroughly. Transfer to an 8-ounce glass mason jar and seal the jar with a tight-fitting lid. Label and date the jar.

2. To prepare the tea, place 1 to 2 teaspoons herb mix into a tea strainer or loose-leaf tea bag and into a mug (or place the mix directly in the mug). Pour 10 ounces just-boiled water over the herbs, cover, and let steep for 10 minutes. Strain as needed and enjoy.

SUGGESTED USE/DOSAGE

Prepare and drink hot every few hours until the fever breaks. If excess sweating occurs, take a break and hydrate so as not to bring on exhaustion.

WARNING *Fenugreek is contraindicated for pregnancy. Do not give to children under 5 years of age.*

HEADACHES AND MIGRAINES

Headaches can be caused by any number of physical and environmental triggers, including muscle tension, allergies, or injury. If you are a migraine sufferer who takes prescription medication and want to try an herbal remedy, please set up a care plan for yourself first. And keep in touch with your healthcare provider to make sure there are no contraindications between your prescription medication and any herbs you might use.

Migraine-Relief Tincture

YIELDS 8 FLUID OUNCES (480 DOSES)

Living with migraines can be intensely stressful. You never know when you will be knocked down by pain, light sensitivity, nausea, and dizziness. The herbs in this recipe have been used to stave off headaches and migraines for generations (in fact, aspirin was originally derived from white willow). Take your time and be gentle with yourself as you experiment with this tincture. May it bring you reduced pain and fewer instances of migraines.

INGREDIENTS*

¼ **cup feverfew leaf**

¼ **cup white willow bark**

¼ **cup skullcap leaf**

2 **tablespoons rosemary leaf**

2 **tablespoons milky oat tops**

1 **tablespoon lavender flower**

1 **cup 80-proof vodka**

*Ingredients are dried unless otherwise indicated.

INSTRUCTIONS

1. In a 16-ounce glass mason jar, combine all the herbs. Pour in the vodka, seal the jar with a tight-fitting lid, and shake gently. Place the jar in a cool, dark, dry place for 6 to 8 weeks, shaking it every day or two.

2. Strain the tincture through a fine-mesh strainer set over a bowl and use a funnel to transfer it into one amber glass dropper bottle and amber glass tincture bottles with twist caps. Label and date the bottles.

SUGGESTED USE/DOSAGE

Take 10 drops of tincture with water at the first sign or symptoms of a migraine. Take 5 to 10 drops with water every 2 hours for acute conditions and 5 to 10 drops 3 times a day for more chronic conditions. Pay attention to how your body responds and increase the dose slowly.

Headache-Ease Tincture

YIELDS 8 FLUID OUNCES (240 TO 480 DOSES)

Comfort and pain relief is the name of this game, and this remedy aims to bring both. Containing herbs that reduce inflammation and pain while also easing anxiety, this tincture will help you get back in the swing of things in no time.

INGREDIENTS*

¼ **cup skullcap leaf**

¼ **cup passionflower leaf**

2 **tablespoons ginger root**

2 **tablespoons German chamomile flower**

2 **tablespoons lemon balm leaf**

2 **teaspoons rose petals or buds**

¼ **cup cramp bark**

1 **cup 80-proof vodka**

*Ingredients are dried unless otherwise indicated.

INSTRUCTIONS

1. In a 16-ounce glass mason jar, combine all the herbs. Pour in the vodka, seal the jar with a tight-fitting lid, and shake gently. Place the jar in a cool, dark, dry place for 6 to 8 weeks, shaking it once every day or two.

2. Strain the tincture through a fine-mesh strainer set over a bowl and use a funnel to transfer it into one amber glass dropper bottle and amber glass tincture bottles with twist caps. Label and date the bottles.

SUGGESTED USE/DOSAGE

Take ½ to 1 dropperful (½ to 1 mL) twice a day as needed, or add to 1 cup cold or room-temperature water.

WARNING *Do not take if you are pregnant, nursing, have a bleeding disorder, or take blood thinners or sedative medications. Do not give to children under 12 years of age. Avoid lemon balm if you have a sensitive thyroid or hypothyroidism. Be mindful if you are allergic to plants in the Asteraceae and/or Compositae families as chamomile could trigger an allergic reaction.*

INFLAMED AND IRRITATED SKIN

Skin is our largest, most regenerative, and, occasionally, most sensitive organ. It is exposed to endless battering, chemicals, and environmental influence (wind, pollen, sun). For the most part, our skin handles everything we throw at it without a hitch or complaint. And sometimes, when it has had enough, our skin cries out (in the form of rashes, eczema, tightness, and cracking) and it is our job to stop and nourish this beautiful organ that, quite literally, holds us together.

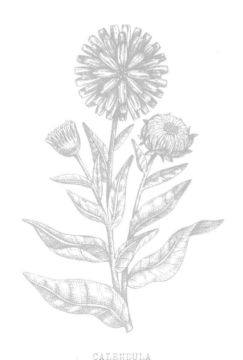

CALENDULA

Derma-Soothe Body Butter

YIELDS 6 OUNCES

If you are anything like me, you often deal with contact dermatitis and just plain dry skin. Having a soothing body butter to ease the itch and heal the dryness is my happy place. This simple, effective body butter is crafted from herbs that help the body heal dryness and itchy patches while also leaving behind soft, happy skin.

INGREDIENTS*

½ **cup plus 2 tablespoons extra-virgin olive oil**

½ **cup calendula flower**

½ **cup plantain leaf**

2 **tablespoons beeswax pellets**

2 **tablespoons shea butter**

Ingredients are dried unless otherwise indicated.

INSTRUCTIONS

1. In a double boiler over low heat, combine the olive oil, calendula, and plantain. Heat for 1 hour to infuse the oil.

2. Place a fine-mesh strainer over a heatproof bowl and line the strainer with cheesecloth. Pour the warm infusion into the cheesecloth, letting the oil strain through. Squeeze the cheesecloth over the strainer to extract all the oil infusion.

3. Add the beeswax pellets and shea butter to the strained oil infusion and place the bowl over the double boiler over low heat. Warm, stirring and watching constantly, until the mixture is melted and combined. Do not let it boil. Immediately pour the melted oil into two 3-ounce glass mason jars. Let sit, untouched, for 3 to 4 hours, or until the oils have set and solidified. Cover and label the jars.

SUGGESTED USE/DOSAGE

Rub the body butter onto affected areas as often as needed.

WARNING *Topical applications containing calendula are considered safe during pregnancy and while nursing, but avoid the chest area so nurslings do not unintentionally ingest any salve.*

Rosacea-Soothing Cream

YIELDS 6 OUNCES

Rosacea is an inflammation of facial skin that causes redness, puffiness, pus-filled pimples, rashes, and pain. There's no single cause, but some outbreak triggers are stress, extreme cold or heat, spicy foods, and alcohol. This cream remedy is created with herbs that contain essential fatty acids and antioxidants as well as nourishing properties to help protect and nurture skin.

INGREDIENTS*

½ **cup jojoba oil**

¼ **cup lavender flower**

¼ **cup green tea leaf**

2 **tablespoons German chamomile**

1 **tablespoon shea butter**

1 **tablespoon cocoa butter**

⅓ **cup pure aloe vera gel**

¼ **cup black cumin seed oil**

*Ingredients are dried unless otherwise indicated.

INSTRUCTIONS

1. In a double boiler over low heat, combine the jojoba oil, lavender, green tea, and chamomile. Heat for 1 hour to infuse the oil.

2. Place a fine-mesh strainer over a heatproof bowl and line the strainer with cheesecloth. Pour the warm infusion into the cheesecloth, letting the oil strain through. Squeeze the cheesecloth over the strainer to extract all the oil infusion.

3. Add the shea butter and cacao butter to the strained oil infusion and place the bowl over the double boiler over low heat. Warm, stirring and watching constantly, until the mixture is melted and combined. Do not let it boil.

4. Remove from the heat and gently stir in the aloe vera gel and black cumin seed oil. Place the oil into the refrigerator to cool slightly, 2 to 4 minutes.

5. Using an immersion blender, blend for 1 to 2 minutes until well mixed and creamy. Alternatively, use a standard blend or handheld mixer to blend. Pour the cream into two 3-ounce glass mason jars. Let sit, untouched, for 3 to 4 hours, or until the oils have set and solidified. Cover and label the jars.

SUGGESTED USE/DOSAGE

Rub the cream onto the affected areas as often as needed.

Flare Cooling Mist

YIELDS 4 FLUID OUNCES

When rosacea flares happen, the skin on your face can feel hot, tight, and uncomfortable. This cooling mist will help calm the flare and soothe away the heat and discomfort. Note, if you have access to aloe plants, use fresh aloe instead of store-bought gel—but please do not pick a plant at random if you are unsure, as some succulents have a similar appearance to aloe but are not safe to use.

INGREDIENTS

½ **cup distilled water**

2 tablespoons lavender flower tincture

2 tablespoons German chamomile flower tincture

1 tablespoon pure aloe vera gel

INSTRUCTIONS

1. In a small bowl, stir together the water, tinctures, and aloe vera gel (if using fresh aloe, push it through a fine-mesh strainer into the bowl).

2. Strain the mixture through a fine-mesh strainer into a measuring cup and use a funnel to transfer it into a 4-ounce amber glass spray bottle. Label and date the bottle.

SUGGESTED USE/DOSAGE

Shake gently before use. Mist onto your face (eyes closed) when you feel a rosacea flare coming on, as often as you wish!

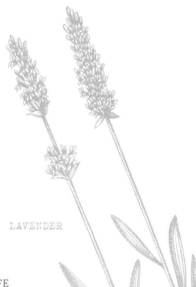

LAVENDER

INSOMNIA

Insomnia can wreak havoc on your mental, emotional, and physical health. Sleep disruption and inadequate sleep can lead to high blood pressure, heart health decline, lack of mental clarity, emotional outbursts, and poor decision making. Lifestyle shifts, such as decreasing screen time, engaging in low-stimuli activities before bed, doing calming movements (such as stretching or yoga and meditation), and eating healthy, easy-to-digest foods (especially for your evening meal) can help improve your sleep/wake rhythms. Adding herbal remedies to your insomnia care plan can help you get your sleep back in order and allow you to have peace of mind and body.

Sound Sleep Tea

YIELDS 14 TABLESPOONS HERB MIX (FOR 21 CUPS OF TEA)

Getting a solid night of sound sleep is necessary for a healthy balanced you. This remedy relies on herbal allies that cause drowsiness, entrain the circadian rhythms, and act as sedatives while also gently calming the mind and body. Be lulled to rest by these helpful herbs and sleep deeply.

INGREDIENTS*

¼ **cup lavender flower**

¼ **cup chamomile flower**

¼ **cup nettles leaf**

2 **tablespoons hops flower**

*Ingredients are dried unless otherwise indicated.

INSTRUCTIONS

1. In a small bowl, stir together all the herbs until mixed thoroughly. Transfer to an 8-ounce glass mason jar and seal the jar with a tight-fitting lid. Label and date the jar.

2. To prepare the tea, place 2 teaspoons herb mix into a tea strainer or loose-leaf tea bag and into a mug (or place the mix directly in the mug). Pour 1 cup just-boiled water over the herbs, cover, and let steep for 10 minutes. Strain as needed.

SUGGESTED USE/DOSAGE

Drink 1 cup at least 1 hour before bedtime.

WARNING *Avoid nettles leaf if you are pregnant, nursing, or taking blood pressure medication. Be mindful if you are allergic to plants in the Asteraceae and/or Compositae families as chamomile could trigger an allergic reaction.*

Rest Well Tincture

YIELDS 2 FLUID OUNCES (20 DOSES)

A good night's sleep is an amazing gift to someone who deals with constant sleep disruption and insomnia. This tincture is crafted from herbs with sedative, nerve-nourishing, anti-anxiety, and naturally calming properties that can help you fall asleep with ease so you get the rest you need.

INGREDIENTS*

2 teaspoons ashwagandha root
1 teaspoon California poppy flower and leaf
1 teaspoon chamomile flower
1 teaspoon nettles leaf
1 teaspoon lemon balm leaf
¼ cup 80-proof vodka

Ingredients are dried unless otherwise indicated.

INSTRUCTIONS

1. In an 8-ounce glass mason jar, combine all the herbs. Pour in the vodka, seal the jar with a tight-fitting lid, and shake gently. Place the jar in a cool, dark, dry place for 4 to 6 weeks, shaking it every day or two.

2. Strain the tincture through a fine-mesh strainer set over a bowl and use a funnel to transfer it into a 2-ounce amber glass dropper bottle. Label and date the bottle.

SUGGESTED USE/DOSAGE

Take 2 dropperfuls (2 mL) at least 30 minutes before bedtime and 1 dropperful (1 mL) when you lie down to go to sleep, or add to 1 cup cold or room-temperature water.

WARNING *Avoid lemon balm if you have a sensitive thyroid or hypothyroidism. Avoid nettles leaf if you are pregnant, nursing, or taking blood pressure medication. Be mindful if you are allergic to plants in the Asteraceae and/or Compositae families as chamomile could trigger an allergic reaction.*

JOINT INFLAMMATION AND BACK PAIN

Whether caused by diet, physical behaviors, illness, age, or something else entirely, joint pain and inflammation make doing basic tasks a huge chore. By bringing down inflammation and addressing pain points, these remedies can help alleviate pain and get the spring back in your step.

Anti-Inflammation Capsules

YIELDS 120 CAPSULES (60 TO 120 DOSES)

Inflammation is not only one of the most common causes of pain, but also the gateway to illness in the body. The anti-inflammatory powerhouses in this herbal remedy are widely recognized. They are also antioxidative and can even reduce swelling.

INGREDIENTS

½ **cup turmeric powder**

¼ **cup ginger powder**

3 **tablespoons rosemary leaf powder**

1 **tablespoon freshly ground black pepper**

120 **empty size 00 capsules**

INSTRUCTIONS

1. Cover your work surface with a towel.

2. In a medium bowl, stir together all the herbs until mixed thoroughly.

3. Place a tray in the center of the work area and set the bowl of herb powder on the tray. Gather your capsules and an 8-ounce glass mason jar for storing the filled capsules.

4. Working one at a time, open a capsule and use the long side of the capsule to scoop powder into the capsule, pushing it in and pressing it with your finger. When the capsule is full, place the other end of the capsule on and push it down to close. Rub a small amount of the herb remedy onto the outside of the capsule before putting it into the jar. This allows your body to know what it is ingesting and prepare itself to digest and utilize the remedy. Seal the jar with a tight-fitting lid.

SUGGESTED USE/DOSAGE
Take 1 to 2 capsules a day.

WARNING *Do not take if you are allergic to black pepper. Ginger should not be taken by people who have a bleeding disorder or are taking blood thinners. Do not take turmeric if you have liver or bile duct disorders.*

NERVE PAIN AND NEUROPATHY

For some people, nerve pain manifests in sharp, shooting pains that can be intermittent or constant. This is known as neuralgia. For others, the pain manifests more as numbness with tingling, like losing sensation in a limb momentarily—think pins and needles but more intense. This is often associated with nerve impingement (such as sciatica, nerve entrapment, and carpal tunnel syndrome). Using herbal remedies alongside physical therapies and other care programs can help diminish and potentially alleviate nerve pain.

Neuropathy-Ease Tincture

YIELDS 4 FLUID OUNCES (40 DOSES)

Neuropathic numbness and tingling can come from illness as well as from injury. Helping support and nourish your nervous system will assist in bringing about healing that can ease or even stop neuropathic discomforts. This remedy contains herbs that have analgesic, anti-inflammatory, and nerve-supporting properties.

INGREDIENTS*

2 teaspoons nettles leaf
1 teaspoon feverfew leaf
1 teaspoon passionflower leaf
1 teaspoon oatstraw leaf
½ cup 80-proof vodka

*Ingredients are dried unless otherwise indicated.

INSTRUCTIONS

1. In an 8-ounce glass mason jar, combine all the herbs. Pour in the vodka, seal the jar with a tight-fitting lid, and shake gently. Place the jar in a cool, dark, dry place for 6 to 8 weeks, shaking it every 1 to 2 days.

2. Strain the tincture through a fine-mesh strainer set over a bowl and use a funnel to transfer it into one amber glass dropper bottle and amber glass tincture bottles with twist caps. Label and date the bottles.

SUGGESTED USE/DOSAGE

Take 1 dropperful (1 mL) 3 times a day for 8 to 12 weeks, or add to 1 cup cold or room-temperature water.

WARNING *Avoid nettles leaf and passionflower leaf if you are pregnant, nursing, or taking blood pressure medication.*

Neuralgia Pain Tincture

YIELDS 4 FLUID OUNCES (40 DOSES)

Neuralgia pain can be highly disruptive, popping up at random times like an electric shock. Nourishing your nervous system can help limit the occurrences or even stop them in their tracks. This herbal remedy is filled with nervines that help calm nerve pain, ease tension, and relieve inflammation.

INGREDIENTS*

2 teaspoons German chamomile flower
1 teaspoon oatstraw leaf
1 teaspoon skullcap leaf
1 teaspoon lemon balm leaf
½ cup 80-proof vodka

Ingredients are dried unless otherwise indicated.

INSTRUCTIONS

1. In an 8-ounce glass mason jar, combine all the herbs. Pour in the vodka, seal the jar with a tight-fitting lid, and shake gently. Place the jar in a cool, dark, dry place for 6 to 8 weeks, shaking it every 1 to 2 days.

2. Strain the tincture through a fine-mesh strainer set over a bowl and use a funnel to transfer it into one amber glass dropper bottle and amber glass tincture bottles with twist caps. Label and date the bottles.

SUGGESTED USE/DOSAGE

Take 1 dropperful (1 mL) 3 times a day for 8 to 12 weeks, or add to 1 cup cold or room-temperature water.

WARNING *Avoid lemon balm if you have a sensitive thyroid or hypothyroidism. Do not take if you are pregnant or take sedative medications. Be mindful if you are allergic to plants in the Asteraceae and/or Compositae families as chamomile could trigger an allergic reaction.*

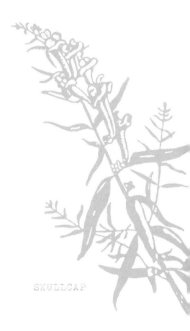

SKULLCAP

Managing Respiratory Illnesses and Allergies

Breathing with ease is something people often take for granted until they cannot do it. With higher pollen counts, gustier winds, and warmer, drier days due to climate change, more and more people have breathing difficulties and respiratory inflammation leading to asthmatic behaviors. Although we might not be able to fully control the environment around us, we can mitigate how our body reacts to triggers that affect our well-being.

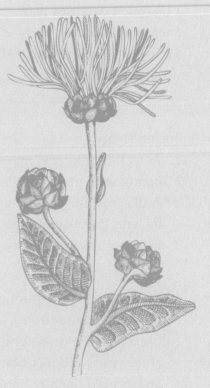

ELECAMPANE

ASTHMA AND WHEEZING

Asthma is an inflammatory reaction of the body that is most often hereditary in nature. It can be triggered by stress, dust, chemical scents, or even cold air. Although asthma is a systemic disruption, there are herbs that can help soothe the bronchial inflammation and associated wheezing and discomfort that goes along with it.

Asthma-Aid Tincture

YIELDS 4 FLUID OUNCES (120 DOSES)

The tightness of asthma caused by bronchial inflammation can create discomfort and anxiety as you try to catch your breath and breathe more easily. The herbs in this remedy help combat inflammation, calm the respiratory nerves, and diminish coughing while helping soothe the airways.

INGREDIENTS*

2 tablespoons wild cherry bark
2 tablespoons licorice root
1 tablespoon elecampane root
1 tablespoon plantain leaf
½ cup 80-proof vodka

Ingredients are dried unless otherwise indicated.

INSTRUCTIONS

1. In an 8-ounce glass mason jar, combine all the herbs. Pour in the vodka, seal the jar with a tight-fitting lid, and shake gently. Place the jar in a cool, dark, dry place for 6 to 8 weeks, shaking it every 1 to 2 days.

2. Strain the tincture through a fine-mesh strainer set over a bowl and use a funnel to transfer it into one amber glass dropper bottle and amber glass tincture bottles with twist caps. Label and date the bottles.

SUGGESTED USE/DOSAGE

Take 1 dropperful (1 mL) as needed for cough associated with asthma, or add to 1 cup cold or room-temperature water.

WARNING *If you take blood thinners, consult your doctor before use. Be mindful if you are allergic to plants in the Asteraceae and/or Compositae families as elecampane could trigger an allergic reaction.*

BRONCHIAL INFLAMMATION AND COUGH

Bronchial inflammation can be caused by illness (such as a viral or upper-respiratory infection), environmental particulates (such as wildfire smoke, smog and other air pollution, cigarette smoke, and vehicle exhaust), or systemic disruption where inflammation is involved. Supporting your respiratory system using herbal remedies and treatments will help you maintain healthy bronchia and easier breathing.

Bronchial Support Syrup

YIELDS ABOUT 32 OUNCES (192 DOSES)

The barking cough and tightness that accompanies bronchial inflammation can be painful. This delicious herbal syrup contains herbs that soothe the bronchioles and diminish inflammation.

INGREDIENTS*

8 cups water
¼ cup elecampane root
¼ cup wild cherry bark
½ cup plantain leaf
½ cup marshmallow root
½ cup mullein leaf
3 cups honey, sugar, or glycerite
¼ cup apple cider vinegar

Ingredients are dried unless otherwise indicated.

INSTRUCTIONS

1. In a medium saucepan over high heat, combine the water, elecampane root, and wild cherry bark. Bring to a boil. Reduce the heat to low and simmer the herbs for 30 minutes.

2. Remove the pot from the heat and add the plantain, marshmallow, and mullein. Cover and let steep for 1 hour.

3. Place a fine-mesh strainer over a heatproof bowl and line the strainer with cheesecloth. Pour the herbal liquid into the cheesecloth and let drain.

4. Stir the honey into the drained liquid. Let cool.

5. Stir in the vinegar.

6. Using a funnel, transfer the syrup to two 16-ounce amber glass bottles with twist caps. Seal, label, and date the bottles.

SUGGESTED USE/DOSAGE

Take 1 teaspoon (5 mL) 3 to 4 times a day as needed.

WARNING *If you take any medications, talk to your healthcare provider before using this remedy. Marshmallow root can disrupt the ability of medications to be absorbed.*

Marshmallow has also shown blood sugar-lowering properties, so do not use if you take diabetes medication. Be mindful if you are allergic to plants in the Asteraceae and/or Compositae families as elecampane could trigger an allergic reaction.

Respiratory Support Tea

YIELDS 3 CUPS PLUS 2 TABLESPOONS HERB MIX (FOR 50 CUPS OF TEA)

Using herbal remedies that nourish the respiratory system will help you stay healthier and breathe easier.

INGREDIENTS*

1 cup elecampane root

⅔ cup marshmallow root

⅔ cup mullein leaf

⅓ cup calendula flower

⅓ cup peppermint leaf

2 tablespoons plus 2 teaspoons ginger root

Honey or other natural sweetener, for serving (optional)

Ingredients are dried unless otherwise indicated.

INSTRUCTIONS

1. In a medium bowl, stir together all the herbs until mixed thoroughly. Transfer to a 32-ounce glass mason jar. Label and date the jar.

2. To prepare the tea, place 1 tablespoon herb mix into a tea strainer or loose-leaf tea bag and into a mug (or place the mix directly in the mug). Pour 1 cup just-boiled water over the tea. Cover and let steep for 30 minutes, or up to 1 hour. Strain and sweeten as desired.

SUGGESTED USE/DOSAGE

Drink 1 cup 2 to 4 times a day for up to 3 weeks for acute symptoms. Take a week off and, if necessary, begin the regimen again for another 3 weeks.

WARNING *If you take any medications, talk to your healthcare provider before using this remedy. Marshmallow root can disrupt the ability of medications to be absorbed. Marshmallow has also shown blood sugar-lowering properties, so do not use if you take diabetes medication. Ginger should not be taken by people who have a bleeding disorder or are taking blood thinners. Do not consume calendula if you are pregnant, as it could trigger a miscarriage, or nursing. Do not give to children under 5 years of age. Be mindful, too, if you are allergic to plants in the Asteraceae and/or Compositae families as calendula and elecampane may trigger an allergic reaction. Large doses of elecampane can cause nausea, vomiting, diarrhea, and abdominal cramping.*

CONGESTION (NASAL AND CHEST)

Being unable to breathe with ease can be disconcerting and disruptive. Nasal and sinus congestion can be brought on by environmental triggers, allergies, and inflammation in the body as well as illness. Easing the mucus and inflammation associated with nasal and chest congestion will help bring calm and health back into your life.

De-Congestion Tea

YIELDS HEAPING 5⅓ CUPS HERB MIX (FOR ABOUT 85 CUPS OF TEA)

When your sinuses are stuffy and your nose is vacillating between flowing like a faucet and locked down like Fort Knox, it is time to reach for this herbal remedy. The herbs in this blend help unlock congestion while supporting the body to clear the illness causing it.

INGREDIENTS*

1 cup dried elderberries
1 cup nettles leaf
1 cup peppermint leaf
1 cup ginger root
1 cup fennel seed
⅔ cup eucalyptus leaf (never oil)
⅓ cup whole cloves

Honey or other natural sweetener, for serving (optional)

Ingredients are dried unless otherwise indicated.

INSTRUCTIONS

1. In a large bowl, stir together all the herbs until mixed thoroughly. Transfer to a 64-ounce glass mason jar. Seal the jar with a tight-fitting lid. Label and date the jar.

2. To prepare the tea, place 1 tablespoon herb mix into a tea strainer or loose-leaf tea bag and into a mug (or place the mix directly in the mug). Pour 1 cup just-boiled water over the tea and let steep for up to 10 minutes. Strain and sweeten as desired.

SUGGESTED USE/DOSAGE

Drink 1 to 3 cups a day as needed.

WARNING *Use fennel with caution during pregnancy. Do not give to children under 5 years of age. If giving to older children, eucalyptus must be given in small doses only and monitored in to avoid potential toxicity. Avoid nettles leaf if you are pregnant, nursing, or taking blood pressure medication. Ginger should not be taken by people who have a bleeding disorder or are taking blood thinners.*

Decongestant Chest Rub

YIELDS 16 OUNCES

I can clearly remember being a kid, sick with a chest cold, knowing the chest rub my mom would bring would help me breathe again. This herbal version of that store-bought chest rub contains herbs that act as an expectorant when inhaled, helping clear mucus and phlegm while their naturally antiseptic properties fight off infection.

INGREDIENTS*

½ **cup plus 2 tablespoons extra-virgin olive oil**

1 **tablespoon cocoa butter**

1 **tablespoon shea butter**

¼ **cup eucalyptus leaf**

¼ **cup peppermint leaf**

2 **tablespoons lavender flower**

2 **tablespoons rosemary leaf**

2 **tablespoons beeswax pellets**

*Ingredients are dried unless otherwise indicated.

INSTRUCTIONS

1. In a double boiler over low heat, combine the olive oil, cocoa butter, shea butter, eucalyptus, peppermint, lavender, and rosemary. Heat for 1 hour to infuse the oil.

2. Place a fine-mesh strainer over a heatproof bowl and line the strainer with cheesecloth. Pour the warm infusion into the cheesecloth, letting the oil strain through. Squeeze the cheesecloth over the strainer to extract all the oil infusion.

3. Add the beeswax pellets to the strained oil infusion and place the bowl over the double boiler over low heat. Warm, stirring and watching constantly, until the mixture is melted and combined. Do not let it boil. Immediately pour the melted oil into two 8-ounce glass mason jars. Let sit, untouched, for 3 to 4 hours, or until the oils have set and solidified. Cover and label the jars.

SUGGESTED USE/DOSAGE

Rub onto the chest and/or back as needed.

WARNING *Not safe for children under 10 years of age, as certain volatile oils in the herbs used can cause respiratory distress and difficulty breathing.*

Herbal Decongestant Steam

YIELDS HEAPING 1 CUP HERB MIX (ABOUT 17 STEAMS)

If you are feeling sick, stuffy, and congested, this steam is a great way to start—or end—your day. This remedy includes herbs that help open your airways and allow you to breathe deeply.

INGREDIENTS*

¼ **cup sea salt (do not use iodized salt)**
¼ **cup eucalyptus leaf**
3 tablespoons thyme leaf
2 tablespoons dried orange peel
2 tablespoons peppermint leaf
1 tablespoon whole cloves
1 tablespoon German chamomile flower

Ingredients are dried unless otherwise indicated.

INSTRUCTIONS

1. In a medium bowl, stir together the salt and herbs until mixed thoroughly. Transfer to an 8-ounce glass mason jar and seal the jar with a tight-fitting lid. Label and date the jar.

2. To prepare a steam, in a medium pot, bring 4 to 6 cups of water to a boil over high heat.

3. Grab three towels.

4. Place 1 tablespoon herb mix into a large bowl. Lay a folded towel on a sturdy, hard surface and place the bowl on it. Pour the boiling water over the herbs. Cover the bowl with a second towel and let steep for 5 to 10 minutes.

5. When the remedy is ready, remove the towel and lean over the steam, being careful not to burn yourself. Drape the remaining towel over your head and the bowl, covering any gaping openings so the steam stays trapped under the towel with you. Lean 5 to 10 inches away from the bowl, close your eyes, breathe deeply, and let the steam soothe your lungs, sinuses, eyes, and skin. Steam for no more than 10 minutes in one sitting.

SUGGESTED USE/DOSAGE

You can steam several times a day. Pay attention to how you feel after each steam, especially your breathing, skin, eyes, and sinuses.

WARNING *Do not use with children under 5 years of age.*

CORONAVIRUS/COVID (INCLUDING LONG COVID)

COVID-19 took the world, and our collective health, by storm. It wreaked havoc on every system in the body and left lots of healing to be done in its wake. Years after the initial pandemic, we are still reeling as we deal with each new variant of this disease. Because COVID is a multisystem illness that creates a cascade of disruption within the body, the effort to pin down treatments keeps researchers on their toes. And, for some people, even after the initial virus is gone, long-lasting symptoms linger. These can include:

- ACE2 inhibition
- Brain fog
- Chest pain
- Inflammation throughout the body, especially in the respiratory and digestive systems, nerves, and joints
- Intense fatigue

Herbal remedies can be a part of a long-term plan for wellness and regaining health after COVID.

Rhodiola Root Tea

YIELDS 16 FLUID OUNCES (1 OR 2 DOSES)

Sometimes an herb is so good at what it does that it gets to stand alone. Rhodiola is well known for its immune-supporting properties and, more recently, it's been found to help combat COVID fatigue.

INGREDIENTS

1 tablespoon dried rhodiola root
Honey or other natural sweetener, for serving (optional)

INSTRUCTIONS

In a medium saucepan over medium heat, combine the rhodiola and 2½ cups water. Bring to a simmer, cover the pot, and simmer for 20 to 30 minutes. Strain and sweeten as desired.

SUGGESTED USE/DOSAGE

Drink 1 to 2 cups maximum a day for 6 to 12 weeks. Then, take a break for several weeks.

WARNING *This tea is not suggested for long-term, continuous use.*

ACE2 Receptor Support Tea

YIELDS 16 FLUID OUNCES (1 OR 2 DOSES)

COVID-19 damages our body's ACE2 receptors (regulatory enzymes that exist on the outer layers of cells on certain organs such as the heart and lungs). This remedy incorporates herbal allies known to protect ACE2 receptors.

INGREDIENTS*

2 tablespoons skullcap leaf

2 tablespoons elderflower

1 tablespoon licorice root

1 tablespoon elecampane root

Honey or other natural sweetener, for serving (optional)

*Ingredients are dried unless otherwise indicated.

INSTRUCTIONS

In a medium saucepan over medium heat, combine the herbs and 2½ cups water. Bring to a simmer, cover the pot, and simmer for 20 to 30 minutes. Strain and sweeten as desired.

SUGGESTED USE/DOSAGE

Drink 1 to 2 cups a day for 6 to 12 weeks. Then, take a break for several weeks.

WARNING *Do not take if you are pregnant or take sedative medications. Be mindful if you are allergic to plants in the Asteraceae and/or Compositae families as elecampane could trigger an allergic reaction.*

Astragalus Root Chicken Soup

YIELDS 8 CUPS

Long COVID is the persistent systemic immune response to exposure to the SARS-CoV-2 virus, otherwise known as COVID-19. I have lived with long COVID, and its cascade of systemic destruction and healing, for more than three years. Finding herbs that actually help my body heal has been a game changer! Astragalus is one of them; it has fantastic antiviral properties and provides strong immune system support.

INGREDIENTS

1 small whole chicken, rinsed inside and out

1 head garlic

2 large white onions

1 (2- to 3-inch) piece fresh ginger, cut into ½-inch pieces

1 bundle fresh rosemary (1 to 2 ounces)

1 bundle fresh nettles (1 to 2 ounces)

5 slices dried astragalus root

1 bunch celery, chopped

1 tablespoon sea salt (or to taste)

1½ teaspoons freshly ground black pepper (or to taste; omit if you are allergic)

INSTRUCTIONS

1. Place the whole chicken, skin on, in a large soup pot.

2. Halve the garlic head, leaving the skins on, and add the garlic to the pot.

3. Quarter the onions, leaving the skins on, and add to the pot. Add the ginger.

4. Using kitchen twine, tie the rosemary bundle and nettles bundle together at the stem ends and place them in the pot along with the astragalus.

5. Fill the pot two-thirds full of water, making sure the chicken is fully submerged, and bring to a boil over high heat. Reduce the heat to maintain a simmer and cook for 1 to 2 hours, or until the chicken is cooked all the way through (165°F on a meat thermometer) and the meat is falling off the bone.

   Remove the pot from the heat and let the soup cool slightly.

6. Using tongs, transfer the chicken to a cutting board. When cool enough to handle, shred the chicken from the bones, discarding the bones. Chop the skin if desired, or discard, and set aside.

7. Place a large fine-mesh strainer over a large heatproof bowl and carefully pour the broth into the strainer. Remove any skin and the herb bundle.

8. Push the garlic through the strainer to create a paste and let it fall into the broth. Remove the skins from the onions, break the onions apart, and put them into the broth. Discard any remaining solids.

9. Add the celery to the broth, along with the shredded chicken and skin (if using). Taste and season as needed with salt and pepper.

SUGGESTED USE/DOSAGE

Eat as much of this yummy soup as you want.

WARNING *Avoid nettles leaf if you are pregnant, nursing, or taking blood pressure medication. Ginger should not be taken by people who have a bleeding disorder or are taking blood thinners.*

SINUS INFECTIONS AND RHINOSINUSITIS

Rhinosinusitis is persistent inflammation of the sinus cavity, often (though not always) caused by some sort of environmental trigger. Sinus infections and rhinosinusitis have similar behaviors—inflaming the sinuses, causing pain, and making it difficult to breathe. When the stuffiness, headache, and inflammation hit, it can feel like your head is filled with sand. Herbal rinses, teas, and other remedies can help bring down the inflammation, clear the sinuses, and get you breathing well again.

Sinusitis-Relief Tea

YIELDS 1 CUP HERB MIX (FOR 24 TO 48 CUPS OF TEA)

Sinusitis can make it difficult to breathe and cause puffiness in and around the eyes and nose due to the inflammation it creates. The anti-inflammatory and anti-allergy properties of the herbs in this remedy allow you to find ease and be able to take a deep breath.

INGREDIENTS*
¼ **cup lemon peel**
¼ **cup nettles leaf**
¼ **cup elderflower**
2 **tablespoons thyme leaf**
2 **tablespoons marshmallow root**
Honey or other natural sweetener, for serving (optional)

Ingredients are dried unless otherwise indicated.

INSTRUCTIONS

1. In a small bowl, stir together all the herbs until mixed thoroughly. Transfer to an 8-ounce glass mason jar and seal the jar with a tight-fitting lid. Label and date the jar.

2. To prepare the tea, place 1 to 2 teaspoons herb mix into a tea strainer or loose-leaf tea bag and into a mug (or place the mix directly in the mug). Pour 10 ounces just-boiled water over the herbs, cover, and let steep for 10 minutes. Strain as needed. Sweeten if desired and enjoy.

SUGGESTED USE/DOSAGE
Drink 1 cup a day as symptoms persist, sipped throughout the day.

WARNING *If you take any medications, talk to your healthcare provider before using this remedy, including for hypertension. Marshmallow root can disrupt the ability of medications to be absorbed. Marshmallow has also shown blood sugar–lowering properties, so do not use if you take diabetes medication. Avoid nettles leaf if you are pregnant, nursing, or taking blood pressure medication.*

Herbal Sinus Rinse

YIELDS 32 FLUID OUNCES (FOR 2 RINSES)

Sometimes our sinuses get aggravated from breathing in all the pollen, dust, and random particles in the air as we go about our day. This rinse will help remove any foreign bits bothering your sinuses, as it also helps ease inflammation and congestion.

INGREDIENTS

½ **to 1 teaspoon fine sea salt (not coarse, as large chunks in your nose are painful)**

4 cups boiled water (preferably filtered water)

10 to 20 drops ginger tincture

10 to 20 drops mullein tincture

10 to 20 drops plantain tincture

10 to 20 drops German chamomile tincture

INSTRUCTIONS

1. In a heatproof bowl, combine the salt (but not too much; the water should be no saltier than your tears) and boiled water. As the water cools, add the tinctures.

2. Pour 1 cup of the rinse into your neti pot (fill the pot), a tea pot, or other clean receptacle.

3. Standing in front of a sink, lean over the basin, tilt your head sideways, and slowly pour the rinse into your upper nostril, letting it flow out of your lower nostril. This can cause you to cough, or even gag, as the rinse moves the mucus and other particulates around. This is normal.

4. Refill the pot and repeat on the other side. Gently blow your nose if needed.

SUGGESTED USE/DOSAGE

Use 1 to 3 times a day when other remedies need a boost. Do not use this or any sinus rinse for longer than 2 weeks at a time as persistent use of a nasal rinse can disrupt and clear away too much of the beneficial bacteria in your nose, creating space for more infections to move in.

WARNING *If you take blood thinners, consult your doctor before use.*

Supporting Sexual and Reproductive Health

The health and equilibrium of your sexual and reproductive system affects the balance of your entire body. It works hand in hand with the circulatory system, the nervous system, and the endocrine system. If your sexual and reproductive system is out of whack, your entire body is most likely out of whack in subtle or large ways. Many people seek out allopathic care and Western medications and therapies to "fix" the problems they face, but many of these problems can benefit from holistic and herbal care as well. Adding herbal remedies to sexual and reproductive wellness management is a great way to build personal awareness of your body and its rhythms while helping to bring these systems back into balance.

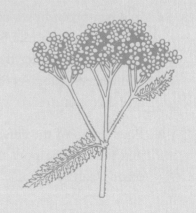

YARROW

MENSTRUAL DISORDERS

Menstrual disorders have become ever more commonplace. Menstruation can be negatively affected by illness, medications, stress, genetics, and hormonal imbalances. Menstrual disorders can manifest with an array of symptoms, such as:

- Body aches
- Complete absence of bleeding or excessive bleeding
- Dizziness
- Mental and emotional disorder (even dysphoria)
- Nausea
- Painful cramps

Bringing herbal remedies into your menstrual healthcare practice will help you manage symptoms and potentially prevent them before they pop up.

Amenorrhea-Aid Tincture

YIELDS 8 FLUID OUNCES (240 DOSES)

Amenorrhea is the absence of menstrual periods. This herbal tincture is made with gentle herbs that, throughout history, have helped restore menstrual flow and regulate the menstrual cycle.

INGREDIENTS*

⅓ **cup fennel seed**

⅓ **cup lemon balm leaf**

⅓ **cup fenugreek**

1 **cup 80-proof vodka**

Ingredients are dried unless otherwise indicated.

INSTRUCTIONS

1. Grind the fennel seeds and put them into a 16-ounce glass mason jar. Add the lemon balm and fenugreek. Pour in the vodka, seal the jar with a tight-fitting lid, and shake gently. Place the jar in a cool, dark, dry place for 6 to 8 weeks, shaking it every day or two.

2. Strain the tincture through a fine-mesh strainer set over a bowl and use a funnel to transfer it into amber glass tincture bottles. Label and date the bottles.

SUGGESTED USE/DOSAGE

Take 1 dropperful (1 mL) a day, or add to 1 cup cold or room-temperature water. Keep track of how your body responds to this remedy. All of these herbs are gentle so you can increase the dose to 2 dropperfuls if needed.

WARNING *Do not use during pregnancy. Avoid lemon balm if you have a sensitive thyroid or hypothyroidism.*

Dysmenorrhea-Relief Tea

YIELDS 1½ CUPS HERB MIX

(FOR 24 CUPS OF TEA)

Dysmenorrhea is pain during the menstrual cycle. My least favorite part of menstruation was the severe, drop-you-to-your-knees cramps I would get *every* month well into my twenties. Over the years, herbs have been crucial in managing my dysmenorrhea, and now I've nearly rid myself of cramps all together. Dysmenorrhea can have a variety of causes, but with patience and experimentation you can find what works for you.

INGREDIENTS*

¼ **cup meadowsweet**

¼ **cup ginger root**

¼ **cup cramp bark**

¼ **cup red raspberry leaf**

¼ **cup dandelion root**

¼ **cup peppermint leaf**

Honey or other natural sweetener, for serving (optional)

Ingredients are dried unless otherwise indicated.

INSTRUCTIONS

1. In a medium bowl, stir together all the herbs until mixed thoroughly. Transfer to a 16-ounce glass mason jar and cover the jar with a tight-fitting lid. Label and date the jar.

2. To prepare the tea, place 1 tablespoon herb mix into a tea strainer or loose-leaf tea bag and into a mug (or place the mix directly in the mug). Pour 1 cup just-boiled water over the tea and let steep for 5 to 10 minutes. Strain and sweetener as desired.

SUGGESTED USE/DOSAGE

Drink 1 to 2 cups a day, 1 to 2 days before you are set to begin bleeding. At the onset of bleeding, drink as often as needed.

WARNING *Avoid red raspberry leaf if you have any hormone-sensitive conditions, such as cancer, endometriosis, or uterine fibroids. Ginger should not be taken by people who have a bleeding disorder or are taking blood thinners. Do not give to children under 5 years of age.*

Menorrhagia-Aid Infusion

YIELDS 1½ CUPS HERB MIX
(FOR 48 CUPS OF TEA)

Menorrhagia is excessively heavy and prolonged menstrual bleeding. It can be caused by hormonal imbalance, illness, and problems associated with the uterus. Menorrhagia not only drains your body of minerals and iron, which can lead to extreme exhaustion, but also makes it difficult to function in your daily life. The herbs in this remedy help normalize the flow of bleeding while nourishing and toning the uterine muscles.

INGREDIENTS*

¼ **cup dried yarrow leaf and flower**

¼ **cup cinnamon chips**

½ **cup red raspberry leaf**

½ **cup nettles leaf**

Honey or other natural sweetener, for serving (optional)

Ingredients are dried unless otherwise indicated.

INSTRUCTIONS

1. In a medium bowl, stir together all the herbs until mixed thoroughly. Transfer to a 16-ounce glass mason jar and seal the jar with a tight-fitting lid. Label and date the jar.

2. To prepare the tea, place 2 tablespoons herb mix into a 32-ounce glass mason jar. Fill the jar with just-boiled water. Stir to make sure all the herbs are covered with water. Seal the jar and let steep for at least 6 hours, or overnight. Strain and sweeten as desired.

SUGGESTED USE/DOSAGE

Drink 1 to 2 cups a day, 1 to 2 days before you are set to begin bleeding. At the onset of bleeding, drink as often as needed throughout the day for the remainder of your bleeding.

WARNING *If you take blood pressure medications, consult your healthcare provider before using this remedy to avoid potential herb/drug contraindications. Avoid red raspberry leaf if you have any hormone-sensitive conditions, such as cancer, endometriosis, or uterine fibroids. Do not take if pregnant or nursing. Avoid nettles leaf if you are pregnant, nursing, or taking blood pressure medication.*

PREMENSTRUAL SYNDROME (PMS)

PMS . . . three little letters that mean so much! Premenstrual syndrome affects nearly three out of every four menstruating people. It includes myriad symptoms such as anxiety, body aches, cramps, fatigue, nausea, and mood swings that range from mild to severe in their intensity and duration. Herbal remedies to ease PMS symptoms have been used for centuries, long before PMS was classified as a medical condition. Adding herbal treatments to your PMS survival toolkit will help get you through those difficult days.

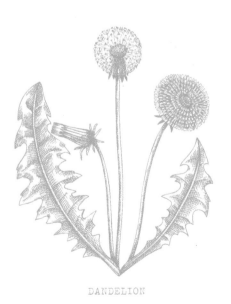

DANDELION

Hormone-Balancing Tea

YIELDS ABOUT 14 TABLESPOONS HERB MIX (FOR 16 CUPS OF TEA)

Your menstrual cycle is ruled by hormones. They signal when eggs should release, when the uterine lining should be shed, and when you should bleed. When these hormones get out of whack, so does your cycle. You can bleed too much or not at all. You can have stressful acne and painful cramps. Staying in balance is the best way to have a smooth cycle. This herbal remedy is crafted from herbs that are known for their hormone-balancing abilities.

INGREDIENTS*

¼ **cup dandelion root**

¼ **cup vitex berries**

2 **tablespoons ginger root**

¼ **cup red raspberry leaf**

Ingredients are dried unless otherwise indicated.

INSTRUCTIONS

1. In a medium bowl, stir together all the herbs until mixed thoroughly. Transfer to an 8-ounce glass mason jar and seal the jar with a tight-fitting lid. Label and date the jar.

2. To prepare the tea, in a small saucepan over medium heat, combine 3 tablespoons herb mix and 4 cups water. Cover the pan and bring to a boil. Turn the heat to low and simmer the tea, covered, for 15 minutes. Remove from the heat, leave covered, and let steep for 20 minutes.

3. Strain and enjoy.

SUGGESTED USE/DOSAGE

Drink 3 to 4 cups a day for 2 weeks. I suggest starting during your follicular phase (right after you stop bleeding), when your body is working to stimulate the release of hormones naturally and encourage follicular activity. Take 1 week off, then repeat the regimen. Keep track of your body's response to the herbs throughout several cycles; take note of changes you notice.

WARNING *Avoid red raspberry leaf if you have any hormone-sensitive conditions, such as cancer, endometriosis, or uterine fibroids. Ginger should not be taken by people who have a bleeding disorder or are taking blood thinners.*

UTERINE LINING DYSFUNCTION

It is estimated that between 70 and 80 percent of uterus-bearers will deal with some form of uterine lining problem by the time they are fifty, including things like uterine polyps, uterine fibroids, and endometriosis. Although these and other uterine disorders are treated with medications and surgery under allopathic medicine, herbal medicinal remedies are an option for gentler, less-invasive first steps of treatment and care.

WARNING *If you take OTC or prescription medications for uterine lining problems, consult your healthcare provider before using these remedies to avoid potential herb/drug contraindications.*

Endo Helper Tea

YIELDS 2⅔ CUPS HERB MIX (FOR ABOUT 10 CUPS OF TEA)

Endometriosis is a dysfunction of the growth and location of the uterine lining. It can cause bloating, pain during intercourse, heavy and irregular cycles, and uterine pain. Often, endometriosis is triggered by an excess of estrogen in the system. This herbal remedy includes herbs that lower estrogen levels, support healthy blood flow, reduce cramping during bleeding, and nourish the uterus.

INGREDIENTS*

1 cup dandelion root

⅔ cup burdock root

⅓ cup chasteberry

⅓ cup ginger root

⅓ cup cinnamon chips

Ingredients are dried unless otherwise indicated.

INSTRUCTIONS

1. In a 32-ounce glass mason jar, combine all the herbs, stir until mixed thoroughly, and seal the jar with a tight-fitting lid. Label and date the jar.

2. To prepare the tea, in a saucepan over low heat, combine ¼ cup herb mix and 4½ cups cold water. Cover the pan with a lid and bring the water to a simmer. Let simmer for 20 minutes, covered.

3. Strain the tea through a fine-mesh strainer into another 32-ounce glass mason jar.

SUGGESTED USE/DOSAGE

Drink 3 to 4 cups a day for 3 to 4 months, allowing time for the herbs to promote the healing process. Keep track of your endometriosis symptoms and whether they diminish or dissipate entirely. Take a break from this remedy at the end of the 3 to 4 months and allow your body to rest. If symptoms return or the diminished symptoms increase, start the remedy again. Stay in communication you're your healthcare professional regarding your endometriosis care.

WARNING *Ginger should not be taken if you have a bleeding disorder or take blood thinners. If you take blood pressure medications, consult your healthcare provider before using this remedy to avoid potential herb/drug contraindications. Avoid during pregnancy.*

Dandelion Root Tincture

YIELDS 8 FLUID OUNCES (240 DOSES)

Many problems with the uterine lining stem from an imbalance in hormones (estrogen, progesterone, testosterone) responsible for regulating your cycles. It is often difficult for the liver to process and purge the excess hormones. Dandelion is a detox powerhouse that also supports healthy liver function, which can help your body cleanse itself naturally of excess hormones and allow your system to get back into balance naturally.

INGREDIENTS*

¹⁄₃ **cup dandelion root**

¹⁄₃ **cup nettles leaf**

¹⁄₃ **cup burdock root**

1 **cup 80-proof vodka**

*Ingredients are dried unless otherwise indicated.

INSTRUCTIONS

1. In a 16-ounce glass mason jar, combine the herbs. Pour in the vodka, seal the jar with a tight-fitting lid, and shake gently. Place the jar in a cool, dark, dry place for 6 to 8 weeks, shaking it every 1 to 2 days.

2. Strain the tincture through a fine-mesh strainer set over a bowl and use a funnel to transfer it into one amber glass dropper bottle and amber glass tincture bottles with twist caps. Label and date the bottles.

SUGGESTED USE/DOSAGE

Take 1 dropperful (1 mL) 1 to 3 times a day as needed, or add to 1 cup cold or room-temperature water or juice.

WARNING *Dandelion root tincture should not be used by people with gallbladder disorders, gallstones, or bowel blockages. It should also be avoided by people taking diuretics, antidepressants, and other medications, as it can affect how they clear the body. If you take any medications, speak to your healthcare provider before taking this remedy to check for potential herb/drug contraindications.*

Infertility

The inability to get pregnant or maintain pregnancies is known as infertility. Infertility can feel like a solitary struggle, a war with your body. But it doesn't have to be. Herbs have been used for millennia to support the reproductive system and aid fertility. Although no single remedy can guarantee a successful pregnancy, herbal remedies that support uterine health, circulatory health, and hormone balance can help increase your body's fertility naturally.

WARNING *If you take hormones to boost fertility, consult your healthcare provider before using this remedy to avoid potential herb/drug contraindications.*

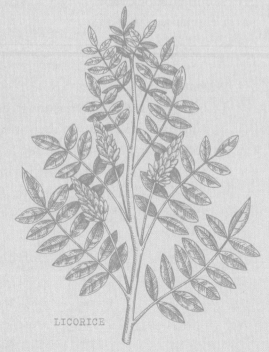

LICORICE

Fertili-Tea

This herbal remedy is filled with fertility-assistive and supportive herbs and plant allies. These herbs are known to help increase ovulation, support the circulatory system, decrease testosterone, and promote uterine health. This delicious tea can assist in your fertility journey.

INGREDIENTS*

⅓ **cup chasteberry**

⅓ **cup ginger root**

⅓ **cup cinnamon chips**

⅓ **cup turmeric root**

1 **cup wild yam root**

½ **cup red clover blossom**

⅔ **cup licorice root**

Ingredients are dried unless otherwise indicated.

INSTRUCTIONS

1. In a medium bowl, stir together all the herbs until mixed thoroughly. Transfer to a 32-ounce glass mason jar. Seal the jar with a tight-fitting lid. Label and date the jar.

2. To prepare the tea, in a medium saucepan over low heat, combine ¼ cup herb mix and 4 cups cold water. Cover the pan and bring the water to a simmer. Let simmer, covered, for 20 minutes.

3. Remove the pan from the heat and let steep for 20 minutes.

4. Strain the tea through a fine-mesh strainer into another 32-ounce glass mason jar.

SUGGESTED USE/DOSAGE

Drink 3 to 4 cups a day. If you believe you have conceived, stop drinking the tea until you know.

WARNING *Ginger should not be taken by people who have a bleeding disorder or are taking blood thinners. If you take blood pressure medications, consult your healthcare provider before using this remedy to avoid potential herb/drug contraindications. Do not take turmeric if you have liver or bile duct disorders. Avoid during pregnancy or nursing.*

Wild Yam Tincture

YIELDS 8 FLUID OUNCES (80 DOSES)

One of the powerhouse herbs used to boost fertility is wild yam, which is known to improve the quality and amount of the cervical mucus that helps sperm successfully make the journey to the egg. Wild yam is also used to help increase and optimize levels of estrogen in the body.

INGREDIENTS*

⅓ **cup wild yam root**

⅓ **cup chasteberry**

1 cup 80-proof vodka

Ingredients are dried unless otherwise indicated.

INSTRUCTIONS

1. In a 16-ounce glass mason jar, combine the herbs. Pour in the vodka, seal the jar with a tight-fitting lid, and shake gently. Place the jar in a cool, dark, dry place for 6 to 8 weeks, shaking it every 1 to 2 days.

2. Strain the tincture through a fine-mesh strainer set over a bowl and use a funnel to transfer it into one amber glass dropper bottle and amber glass tincture bottles with twist caps. Label and date the bottles.

SUGGESTED USE/DOSAGE

Take 60 drops (3 mL) in 1 cup water or juice once a day for up to 12 weeks.

WARNING *Do not take wild yam if you have endometriosis, uterine fibroids, or certain cancers. Wild yam should not be used if you have protein S deficiency without first consulting your healthcare provider.*

Hormone Replacement Therapy

People seek out hormone replacement therapy because their bodies cannot produce the kind of hormone or the amount of hormone needed to keep them in their best health. Hormone therapy can be used to assist in reproductive health as well as gender identity health. Herbal remedies can help the body flush hormones as well as metabolize and utilize hormones more effectively. While herbal remedies are a wonderful part of hormone therapy, they are only one piece in the puzzle. Alongside mental/emotional therapies and other gender-affirming care, herbal remedies can help you have fulfilling and well-rounded HRT care.

WARNING *If you take medications for hormone replacement therapy under the care of a doctor, consult them before taking any herbal remedies to avoid potential herb/drug contraindications.*

NETTLE

Estrogen Therapy Support Tincture

YIELDS 8 FLUID OUNCES (120 TO 240 DOSES)

Estrogen therapy can help a person reach their goals for a healthy, balanced hormone system, but it can occasionally throw other systems out of balance. The herbs in this remedy help the body metabolize estrogen and utilize it efficiently while maintaining harmony gently.

INGREDIENTS*

¼ **cup maca root**

¼ **cup licorice root**

¼ **cup dandelion root**

¼ **cup red reishi mushroom powder**

1 **cup 80-proof vodka**

Ingredients are dried unless otherwise indicated.

INSTRUCTIONS

1. In a 16-ounce glass mason jar, combine the herbs. Pour in the vodka, seal the jar with a tight-fitting lid, and shake gently. Place the jar in a cool, dark, dry place for 6 to 8 weeks, shaking it every 1 to 2 days.

2. Strain the tincture through a fine-mesh strainer lined with cheesecloth and set over a bowl and use a funnel to transfer it into one amber glass dropper bottle and amber glass tincture bottles with twist caps. Label and date the bottles.

SUGGESTED USE/DOSAGE

Take 1 to 2 dropperfuls (1 to 2 mL) 1 to 3 times a day, or add to 1 cup cold or room-temperature water or juice. Pay attention to how your body responds to the remedy and adjust the dose as needed.

WARNING *If you take prescription HRT medications, consult your healthcare provider before using this remedy to avoid potential herb/drug contraindications.*

Testosterone Therapy Support Tincture

YIELDS 8 FLUID OUNCES (120 TO 240 DOSES)

Herbs are a great way to support hormone balance and increase the body's ability to produce the hormones it needs, metabolize hormones effectively, and utilize the hormones present optimally. This remedy uses herbs that have natural testosterone-boosting properties.

INGREDIENTS*

⅓ **cup nettles leaf**

⅓ **cup red clover blossom**

3 tablespoons pine pollen

3 tablespoons ashwagandha root

3 tablespoons fennel seed

3 tablespoons red raspberry leaf

1 cup 80-proof vodka

Ingredients are dried unless otherwise indicated.

INSTRUCTIONS

1. In a 16-ounce glass mason jar, combine the herbs. Pour in the vodka, seal the jar with a tight-fitting lid, and shake gently. Place the jar in a cool, dark, dry place for 6 to 8 weeks, shaking it every 1 to 2 days.

2. Strain the tincture through a fine-mesh strainer lined with cheesecloth and set over a bowl and use a funnel to transfer it into one amber glass dropper bottle and amber glass tincture bottles with twist caps. Label and date the bottles.

SUGGESTED USE/DOSAGE

Take 1 to 2 dropperfuls (1 to 2 mL) 1 to 3 times a day, or add to 1 cup cold or room-temperature water or juice. Pay attention to how your body responds to the remedy, and adjust the dose as needed.

WARNING *If you take prescription HRT medications, consult your healthcare provider before taking this remedy to avoid potential herb/drug contraindications. Avoid red raspberry leaf if you have any hormone-sensitive conditions, such as cancer, endometriosis, or uterine fibroids. Use fennel with caution during pregnancy. Avoid nettles leaf if you are pregnant, nursing, or taking blood pressure medication.*

Decreased Sex Drive

Decreased sex drive is a common disorder that can affect sexually mature adults regardless of age. It can be precipitated by mental and emotional turmoil such as stress, anxiety, or depression as well as physiological disruption, such as issues with the liver or kidneys, or hormone imbalance. Speaking to an allopathic healthcare provider can help you understand the root of the problem, be it mental/emotional or physical. Once you know the root cause, you can work with herbal remedies to help get back your mojo and increase your libido so diminished sex drive is a thing of the past.

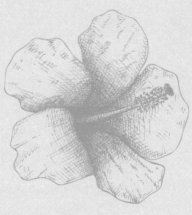

HIBISCUS

Chocolate Love Balls

YIELDS ABOUT TEN 1- TO 2-INCH BALLS

Kicking the libido into gear isn't just about the technical side of things. It's also about being fun and frisky! This recipe is a favorite because it involves chocolate, and creating these treats always makes me feel a little feisty (even before I eat them).

INGREDIENTS

¾ **cup nut or seed butter**

½ **cup tahini**

½ **cup honey**

2 tablespoons cacao powder, plus a small amount for dusting

1 tablespoon maca powder

1 tablespoon shatavari powder

1 tablespoon rose petal powder

1 tablespoon cinnamon powder

1 teaspoon vanilla bean powder (optional)

2 tablespoons mini semisweet chocolate chips (optional)

INSTRUCTIONS

1. Line a plate with parchment paper.

2. In a medium bowl, stir together the nut butter, tahini, and honey.

3. Add the cacao powder, herb powders, and vanilla powder (if using). Stir until well combined.

4. Stir in the chocolate chips (if using). You should have a fairly stiff, rough dough.

5. Roll the dough into 1- to 2-inch balls (I wear food-grade disposable gloves for this) and place them on the prepared plate. Dust the balls with cacao powder. Refrigerate in an airtight container until ready to use. Freeze what you won't eat within 3 to 5 days.

SUGGESTED USE/DOSAGE

A serving is 2 to 4 balls, but enjoy more if you wish.

WARNING *If you take blood pressure medications, consult your healthcare provider before using this remedy to avoid potential herb/drug contraindications. Limit cinnamon use during pregnancy.*

Aphrodisiac Tea

YIELDS SCANT ½ CUP HERB MIX (FOR ABOUT
7 CUPS OF TEA)

Desire isn't a constant. Stress, fatigue, and feeling low can all dampen the desire to engage sexually or intimately. Sometimes, a little help to get the fires burning is all that is needed to turn sexual disinterest into sexual desire. The herbs in this tea not only help increase libido, but also are good for circulation and taste lovely. This is a fun cup to have when you are looking to get intimate with someone special.

INGREDIENTS*

¼ cup rose petals

2 tablespoons damiana leaf

2 teaspoons ginger root

1 teaspoon ashwagandha leaf

1 teaspoon hibiscus flower

1 teaspoon rosehips

**Honey or other natural sweetener, for
    serving (optional)**

Ingredients are dried unless otherwise indicated.

INSTRUCTIONS

1. In a medium bowl, stir together all the herbs until mixed thoroughly. Transfer to an 8-ounce glass mason jar and seal with a tight-fitting lid. Label and date the jar.

2. To prepare the tea, place 1 table-spoon herb mix into a tea strainer or loose-leaf tea bag and into a mug (or place the mix directly in the mug). Pour 1 cup just-boiled water over the tea and let steep for 10 minutes. Strain and sweeten as desired.

SUGGESTED USE/DOSAGE

Drink 1 cup 30 minutes before you plan to get intimate. It can be part of the seduction. Give them a cup, too, and see where the energy carries you!

WARNING *Ginger should not be taken by people who have a bleeding disorder or are taking blood thinners. Avoid hibiscus if pregnant, hypotensive, or you have high blood pressure and take blood pressure medications.*

Erectile Dysfunction

Sexual vitality is an important part of a healthy sex life. The ability to maintain a strong erection is what makes penetrative sexual intercourse with a penis possible. Erectile dysfunction can have physiological causes such as high blood pressure, liver and kidney disorders, low testosterone, and prostate disorders. It can also have mental, emotional, and lifestyle causes such as stress, anxiety, fear of intimate connection, injury, depression, lack of good sleep and nutrition, medications and/or drugs, and alcohol use. Seeking counsel for any mental or emotional needs and improving harmful practices (such as excessive alcohol intake) will go a long way to help increase vitality. Herbal remedies can help move you the rest of the way from an inability to maintain an erection to healthy erectile function.

Ashwagandha and Matcha Latte

The herbs in this remedy boost your ability to have and maintain an erection while increasing libido and sperm count and motility, while decreasing the inflammation that can be a part of erectile dysfunction.

INGREDIENTS

½ **cup hot water**

¼ **to ½ cup oat milk**

1 teaspoon maca powder

1 teaspoon ashwagandha powder

1 teaspoon matcha powder

½ **teaspoon vanilla bean powder (optional)**

Honey or other natural sweetener, for serving

INSTRUCTIONS

1. In a small saucepan over high heat, bring the water to a boil.

2. In another small saucepan over low heat, warm the oat milk.

3. In a mug, combine all the powders, including the vanilla (if using). Add 2 to 3 tablespoons just-boiled water and whisk into a froth until the powders dissolve.

4. Add ¼ cup just-boiled water to the mug.

5. Froth the oat milk and it pour into the mug. Add honey, if desired. Drink and enjoy.

SUGGESTED USE/DOSAGE

Drink 1 to 2 cups a day.

ED-Away Capsules

YIELDS 120 CAPSULES (40 DOSES)

Hormone and systemic support are ways in which you can help heal the problem of erectile dysfunction. The herbs in this remedy are known for improving circulation and heart health, boosting testosterone production, and increasing libido.

INGREDIENTS

2 tablespoons beetroot powder

2 tablespoons fenugreek seed powder

1 tablespoon ashwagandha powder

1 tablespoon maca powder

1 tablespoon shatavari powder

1½ teaspoons ginger powder

1½ teaspoons garlic powder

120 size 00 empty capsules

INSTRUCTIONS

1. Cover your work surface with a towel.

2. In a medium bowl, stir together the herb powders until mixed thoroughly.

3. Place a tray in the center of the work area and set the bowl of herb powder onto the tray. Gather the capsules and an 8-ounce glass mason jar for storing the filled capsules.

4. Working one at a time, open a capsule and use the long side of the capsule to scoop powder into the capsule, pushing it in and pressing it with your finger. When the capsule is full, place the other end of the capsule on and push it down to close. Rub a small amount of the herb remedy onto the outside of the capsule before putting it into the jar. This allows your body to know what it is ingesting and prepare itself to digest and utilize the remedy. Seal the jar with a tight-fitting lid.

SUGGESTED USE/DOSAGE

Take 1 capsule 3 times a day for 12 weeks, then take a break. Keep track of how you feel and any changes you notice.

WARNING *Fenugreek is contraindicated for pregnancy. Ginger should not be taken by people who have a bleeding disorder or are taking blood thinners.*

Menopause/Andropause

As we age, our hormone systems begin to shift away from the task of reproduction and into the work of maintaining our bodies throughout our later years. This shift can be challenging, as our hormones rise and fall erratically. For menopause, this means a steep decline in estrogen and progesterone production as well as a diminishing of follicular activity. For andropause, this means a steep decline in testosterone and an increase in a hormone called sex hormone binding globulin (SHBG), which pulls testosterone out of the bloodstream. At times, the symptoms of menopause (hot flashes, anxiety, mood swings) and of andropause (loss of vitality, diminished muscle tone, depression) can create disruption in your life. Adding herbal remedies to your daily wellness practices can help mitigate unpleasant symptoms of menopause/ andropause and boost your energy to allow you to stay active, happy, and healthy.

MINT

Hot Flash Tincture

YIELDS 2 FLUID OUNCES (30 TO 60 DOSES)

When your "own personal sunrise" is giving you sunburn, calm it down with this hot flash tincture.

INGREDIENTS*

2 teaspoons black cohosh root

1 teaspoon motherwort leaf

1 teaspoon wild yam root

1 teaspoon peppermint leaf

¼ cup 80-proof vodka

Ingredients are dried unless otherwise indicated.

INSTRUCTIONS

1. In an 8-ounce glass mason jar, combine the herbs. Pour in the vodka, seal the jar with a tight-fitting lid, and shake gently. Place the jar in a cool, dark, dry place for 4 weeks, shaking it daily.

2. Strain the tincture through a fine-mesh strainer set over a bowl and use a funnel to transfer it into a 2-ounce amber glass dropper bottle. Label and date the bottle.

SUGGESTED USE/DOSAGE

Take 1 to 2 dropperfuls (1 to 2 mL) as needed, or add to 1 cup cold or room-temperature water.

WARNING *Do not give to children under 5 years of age.*

Balanced Menopause Capsules

YIELDS ABOUT 65 CAPSULES (32 DOSES)

Menopausal hormone fluctuations can leave you feeling depleted. The combination of herbs in this remedy will help you find your balance while also nourishing and supporting your system during this shift.

INGREDIENTS

1 tablespoon chasteberry powder

1 tablespoon kelp powder

1 tablespoon burdock root powder

1½ teaspoons turmeric powder

1½ teaspoons licorice root powder

1½ teaspoons cinnamon powder

65 size 00 empty capsules

INSTRUCTIONS

1. Cover your work surface with a towel.

2. In a medium bowl, stir together all the herbs until mixed thoroughly.

3. Place a tray in the center of the work area and set the bowl of herb powder on the tray. Gather your capsules and an 8-ounce glass mason jar for storing the filled capsules.

4. Working one at a time, open a capsule and use the long side of the capsule to scoop powder into the capsule, pushing it in and pressing

it with your finger. When the capsule is full, place the other end of the capsule on and push it down to close. Rub a small amount of the herb remedy onto the outside of the capsule before putting it into the jar. This allows your body to know what it is ingesting and prepare itself to digest and utilize the remedy. Seal the jar with a tight-fitting lid.

SUGGESTED USE/DOSAGE
Take 2 capsules 2 times a day as needed.

WARNING *If you take blood pressure medications, consult your healthcare provider before using this remedy to avoid potential herb/drug contraindications. Do not take turmeric if you have liver or bile duct disorders. Avoid during pregnancy.*

Andropause-Assist Tincture
YIELDS 8 FLUID OUNCES (120 TO 240 DOSES)

During andropause, energy, muscle mass, and even mental and emotional stability can feel like they are falling apart. The herbal combination in this remedy supports your reproductive and hormone systems during this change and can help you feel like you are back on top.

INGREDIENTS*
2 teaspoons ashwagandha root
2 teaspoons nettles leaf
2 teaspoons fenugreek seed
2 teaspoons astragalus root
2 teaspoons wild yam root
2 teaspoons ginger root
1 cup 80-proof vodka

Ingredients are dried unless otherwise indicated.

INSTRUCTIONS
1. In a 16-ounce glass mason jar, combine all the herbs. Pour in the vodka, seal the jar with a tight-fitting lid and, shake gently. Place the jar in a cool, dark, dry place for 4 weeks, shaking it daily.

2. Strain the tincture through a fine-mesh strainer set over a bowl and use a funnel to transfer it into amber glass tincture bottles. Label and date the bottles.

SUGGESTED USE/DOSAGE
Take 1 dropperful (1 mL) 1 to 2 times a day as needed.

WARNING *Fenugreek is contraindicated for pregnancy. Avoid nettles leaf if you are pregnant, nursing, or taking blood pressure medication. Ginger should not be taken by people who have a bleeding disorder or are taking blood thinners.*

Treating Digestive Issues

As our diets become more complicated by preservatives, processed ingredients, and antibiotic-laden animal products, our digestive systems begin to show ill effects. Leaky gut, irritable bowel syndrome (IBS), Crohn's disease, celiac disease, and gastroesophageal reflux disease (GERD) are just a few of the now very common GI disorders disrupting many lives. Herbal remedies can help support your gastrointestinal system as it works to repair damage and heal.

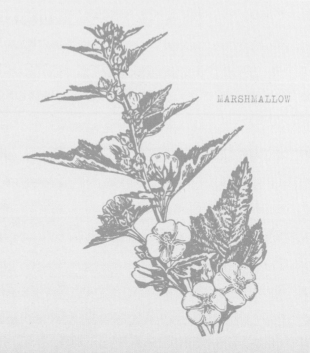

MARSHMALLOW

ACID REFLUX (GERD)

GERD is not just the run-of-the-mill acid reflux we all experience once in a while. It is a disorder marked by chest pain, sour acidic regurgitation, excessive belching, nausea, heartburn, especially after eating, the inability to recline or lie down after eating due to pain and reflux, and difficulty swallowing. This disorder can leave you feeling hungry and exhausted as you seek out foods that won't trigger your disorder. Herbal remedies can help lower the incidence of acidic reflux, decrease GI inflammation, and soothe your digestive system as it heals.

Marshmallow Root Tea

YIELDS ¼ CUP HERB MIX (FOR 4 CUPS OF TEA)

Marshmallow root is a mucilaginous (slimy) herb and, as such, it is wonderfully soothing for inflammation. It has been used to ease the symptoms of GERD as well as other digestive and bowel inflammation problems.

INGREDIENTS

¼ **cup dried marshmallow root**

INSTRUCTIONS

1. This tea is made as a cold infusion. Place the marshmallow root into a 32-ounce glass mason jar and cover with 4 cups cold water.

2. Seal the jar with a tight-fitting lid and refrigerate overnight.

3. Strain.

SUGGESTED USE/DOSAGE

Drink 2 to 8 ounces 1 to 4 times a day as needed.

WARNING *If you take any medications, talk to your healthcare provider before taking marshmallow root as it can disrupt the ability of the medications to be absorbed. Marshmallow has also shown blood sugar–lowering properties, so do not use if you take diabetes medication.*

Golden Milk Latte

YIELDS 2¾ TEASPOONS HERB POWDER (FOR 2 CUPS OF LATTE)

With the gut-soothing properties of oats and the anti-inflammatory properties of turmeric, this palate-pleasing golden milk latte is worthy of a hot cup any time of day.

INGREDIENTS

2 cups oat milk

1 to 2 tablespoons honey or maple syrup (optional)

1 teaspoon turmeric powder

½ teaspoon cinnamon powder

½ teaspoon ginger powder

½ teaspoon nutmeg powder

¼ teaspoon freshly ground black pepper (omit if you are allergic)

INSTRUCTIONS

1. In a saucepan over medium to low heat, warm the oat milk.

2. Whisk in the honey (if using) and herbs so everything is incorporated evenly. Continue to warm for 3 to 4 minutes, whisking occasionally.

3. Remove from the heat and whisk again. Strain as needed into a mug.

SUGGESTED USE/DOSAGE

Drink this latte as often as you desire! I drink at least 1 cup a day during fall and winter, and well into spring, to ease inflammation and because it just tastes so darn good.

WARNING *If you take blood pressure medications, consult your healthcare provider before using this remedy to avoid potential herb/drug contraindications. Ginger should not be taken by people who have a bleeding disorder or are taking blood thinners. Do not take turmeric if you have liver or bile duct disorders. Limit cinnamon use during pregnancy.*

CROHN'S DISEASE

Crohn's disease is not just a gastrointestinal disorder, but also an autoimmune disorder. This means that the body is fighting to function properly on two levels: to digest food functionally and to not attack itself unnecessarily. Symptoms of Crohn's include major abdominal pain, weight loss, diarrhea, and anemia, all directly linked to the body's inability to absorb foods properly. Herbs that are gentle on the system, while also helping rid the body of inflammation and reestablish healthy mucus for the gut lining will nourish the intestinal tract and allow the body to heal.

Inflammation-Ease Tea

YIELDS 5 TEASPOONS HERB MIX (FOR 2 CUPS OF TEA)

When you are having a Crohn's flare, brought on by any number of things (food triggers, stress, infections, diet), the number-one goal is to calm your body and get the symptoms under control. This herbal tea remedy helps protect the lining of the stomach and digestive tract, reduce inflammation, and stimulate the gut's healthy behaviors while allowing the system to heal.

INGREDIENTS*

2 teaspoons marshmallow root

2 teaspoons green tea leaf

1 teaspoon chamomile flower

2 teaspoons honey

Ingredients are dried unless otherwise indicated.

INSTRUCTIONS

1. In a saucepan over medium heat, combine the herbs and 2½ cups water. Bring to a boil.

2. Strain the tea into a large mug and stir in the honey.

SUGGESTED USE/DOSAGE

Drink 1 to 2 cups a day or as needed to ease symptoms. If you take any medications, talk to your healthcare provider before using this remedy.

Marshmallow root can disrupt the ability of medications to be absorbed. Marshmallow has also shown blood sugar–lowering properties, so do not use if you take diabetes medication. Avoid green tea if you take MAOIs (monoamine oxidase inhibitors). Be mindful if you are allergic to plants in the Asteraceae and/or Compositae families as chamomile could trigger an allergic reaction.

Peppermint and Ginger Tincture

YIELDS 2 FLUID OUNCES (30 TO 60 DOSES)

Bowel inflammation can be incredibly painful. It disrupts your life and makes finding safe foods to eat a torturous trial-and-error game. Peppermint's smooth muscle–relaxing properties, combined with the anti-inflammatory and antioxidant properties of ginger bring comfort to aggravated and inflamed bowels.

INGREDIENTS*

2 tablespoons peppermint leaf
2 tablespoons ginger root
¼ cup 80-proof vodka

*Ingredients are dried unless otherwise indicated.

INSTRUCTIONS

1. In an 8-ounce glass mason jar, combine the herbs. Pour in the vodka, cover the jar with a tight-fitting lid, and shake gently. Place the jar in a cool, dark, dry place for 4 to 6 weeks, shaking it every 1 to 2 days.

2. Strain the tincture through a fine-mesh strainer set over a bowl and use a funnel to transfer it into a 2-ounce amber glass dropper bottle. Label and date the bottle.

SUGGESTED USE/DOSAGE

Take 1 to 2 dropperfuls (1 to 2 mL) as needed to ease symptoms, or add to 1 cup cold or room-temperature water.

WARNING *Ginger should not be taken by people who have a bleeding disorder or are taking blood thinners. Do not give to children under 5 years of age.*

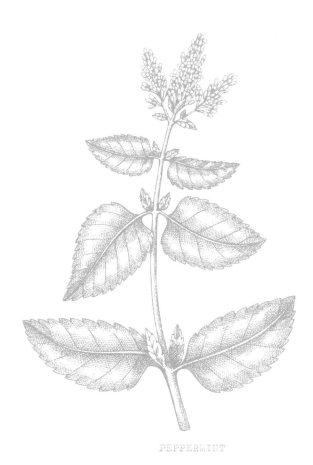

PEPPERMINT

FOOD INTOLERANCE

Food intolerance is the difficulty digesting certain foods. Some of the most common foods that people struggle with are dairy and gluten. Although most food intolerance reactions are mild, some reactions can be debilitating and extremely painful. Gut disorders associated with food intolerance include celiac disease (which like Crohn's is an autoimmune disorder), leaky gut, and irritable bowel syndrome. Herbs that ease symptoms while helping nourish the digestive system and allowing the gut to heal are a great addition to your wellness practice.

Medicinal Herb Pesto

YIELDS ABOUT 4 CUPS

This is one of my favorite recipes. Not only is it crafted from nourishing, gut-healing herbs, but it's also delicious and filled with nutrients.

INGREDIENTS

1½ to 2 cups extra-virgin olive oil

½ cup pumpkin seeds (raw or freshly roasted)

3 or 4 garlic cloves, peeled

1 cup fresh cilantro leaf and stem

½ cup fresh basil leaf

½ cup fresh dandelion leaf

½ cup fresh nettles leaf

2 to 4 tablespoons gluten-free nutritional yeast (nondairy option), or ¼ cup grated parmesan cheese

INSTRUCTIONS

1. In a blender or food processor, combine the olive oil, pumpkin seeds, and garlic. Blend until creamy.

2. A handful at a time, add the greens, blending completely after each addition before adding more. Blend until the pesto is creamy again.

3. Add the nutritional yeast and pulse gently to incorporate. Scrape the pesto out of the blender into four 8-ounce glass mason jars and seal with tight-fitting lids. Keep refrigerated for up to 2 days, or freeze in the jars or portion into ice cube trays for long-term storage.

SUGGESTED USE/DOSAGE

Use this pesto as a treat on your favorite gluten-free pasta, lean protein, crackers, or breads—about ¼ cup equals a serving.

WARNING *Avoid nettles leaf if you are pregnant, nursing, or taking blood pressure medication.*

Celiac-Aid Tincture

YIELDS 4 FLUID OUNCES (60 TO 120 DOSES)

Soothing the inflammation and pain of celiac disease is what this tincture is designed to do. The collection of herbs is anti-inflammatory, aids digestion, and nourishes the digestive system.

INGREDIENTS*

2 tablespoons dandelion root

1 tablespoon chamomile flower

1 tablespoon oatstraw leaf

2 teaspoons marshmallow root

1 teaspoon fenugreek seed

½ cup 80-proof vodka

Ingredients are dried unless otherwise indicated.

INSTRUCTIONS

1. In an 8-ounce glass mason jar, combine the herbs. Pour in the vodka, seal the jar with a tight-fitting lid, and shake gently. Place the jar in a cool, dark, dry place for 6 to 8 weeks, shaking it every 1 to 2 days.

2. Strain the tincture through a fine-mesh strainer set over a bowl and use a funnel to transfer it into one amber glass dropper bottle and amber glass tincture bottles with twist caps. Label and date the bottles.

SUGGESTED USE/DOSAGE

Take 1 to 2 dropperfuls (1 to 2 mL) a day for 12 weeks. Rest for 2 weeks and reassess. Continue as needed.

WARNING *Fenugreek is contraindicated for pregnancy. If you take any medications, talk to your healthcare provider before taking marshmallow root as it can disrupt the ability of the medications to be absorbed. Marshmallow has also shown blood sugar–lowering properties, so do not use if you take diabetes medication. Be mindful if you are allergic to plants in the Asteraceae and/or Compositae families as chamomile could trigger an allergic reaction.*

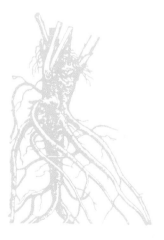

MARSHMALLOW ROOT

IRRITABLE BOWEL SYNDROME

IBS is a multifaceted digestive and gut disorder that can wreak havoc on a person's life. Chronic bouts of diarrhea and/or constipation can make it difficult to be in unfamiliar environments. IBS can be triggered by greasy and fatty foods, lack of fiber, foods made with refined sugars and flours, alcohol, and caffeine as well as stress and anxiety. Crafting remedies that rely on individual herb allies to calm spasms and absorption difficulties—as well as the stress and anxiety that may compound symptoms—can help get your health back on track.

IBS-Ease Tea

YIELDS 14 TABLESPOONS HERB MIX (FOR 21 CUPS OF TEA)

The herbs used to craft this tea are known for their abilities to calm the stomach and intestines while aiding absorption and digestion. This can help ease the spasms, diarrhea, constipation, and pain associated with IBS.

INGREDIENTS*
¼ **cup plantain leaf**
3 **tablespoons ginger root**
3 **tablespoons lemon balm leaf**
2 **tablespoons chamomile flower**
2 **tablespoons peppermint leaf**
Honey or other natural sweetener, for serving (optional)

Ingredients are dried unless otherwise indicated.

INSTRUCTIONS
1. In a medium bowl, stir together all the herbs until mixed thoroughly. Transfer to a 16-ounce glass mason jar and seal the jar with a tight-fitting lid. Label and date the jar.

2. To prepare the tea, place 2 teaspoons herb mix into a tea strainer or loose-leaf tea bag and into a mug (or place the mix directly in the mug). Pour 1 cup just-boiled water over the herbs, cover, and steep for 5 to 10 minutes. Strain and sweeten as desired.

SUGGESTED USE/DOSAGE
Drink 1 to 3 cups a day as needed.

WARNING *Ginger should not be taken by people who have a bleeding disorder or are taking blood thinners. If you take blood thinners, consult your doctor before use. Avoid lemon balm if you have a sensitive thyroid or hypothyroidism. Do not give to children under 5 years of age. Be mindful if you are allergic to plants in the Asteraceae and/or Compositae families as chamomile could trigger an allergic reaction.*

Bowel-Be-Calm Tincture

YIELDS 2 FLUID OUNCES (20 TO 60 DOSES)

When the lining of the stomach and bowel are inflamed and spasming, this tincture can help soothe and calm the disruption and bring things back into balance.

INGREDIENTS

1 teaspoon fennel seed

1 teaspoon turmeric powder

½ teaspoon cinnamon chips

½ teaspoon nutmeg powder

¼ teaspoon freshly ground black pepper (omit if you are allergic)

¼ cup 80-proof vodka

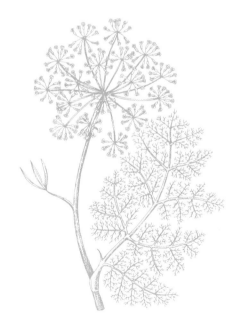

FENNEL

INSTRUCTIONS

1. In an 8-ounce glass mason jar, combine all the herbs. Pour in the vodka, seal the jar with a tight-fitting lid, and shake gently. Place the jar in a cool, dark, dry place for 4 to 6 weeks, shaking it every 1 to 2 days.

2. Strain the tincture through a fine-mesh strainer set over a bowl and use a funnel to transfer it into a 2-ounce amber glass dropper bottle. Label and date the bottle.

SUGGESTED USE/DOSAGE

Take 1 to 3 dropperfuls (1 to 3 mL) once a day, or add to 1 cup cold or room-temperature water. Increase to twice daily if you feel the need for a stronger dose. Pay attention to how your body responds and adjust the dose as needed.

WARNING *If you take blood pressure medications, consult your healthcare provider before using this remedy to avoid potential herb/drug contraindications. Do not take turmeric if you have liver or bile duct disorders. Avoid during pregnancy.*

Support for Chronic Conditions

The occurrence of chronic health conditions has continued to rise year after year. Whether experiencing chronic pain/inflammation or chronic fatigue, many people are unsure about what is causing their daily discomfort and seek ways to bring peace to their days. Dietary and environmental exposure to chemicals known for their inflammatory nature have been associated with many of the symptoms that present in these chronic illnesses. Herbal remedies can help support your body if you are living with chronic health conditions.

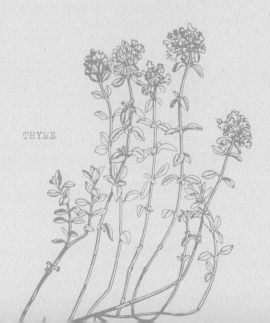

THYME

CHRONIC FATIGUE SYNDROME

Chronic fatigue syndrome (CFS) is more than just feeling really tired. In fact, it is a multisystem neurological disease that stems, in part, from inflammation of the brain and is considered an autoimmune disorder. The root cause of CFS is still unclear, but it is believed that genetics play a key role. Those who suffer from CFS feel exhausted even when they are "well rested" in terms of sleep. Although there is no cure for CFS within allopathic medicine, there are ways to help manage the symptoms. And, of course, herbal remedies have shown positive effects for people living with CFS.

Magnesium Boost Tincture

YIELDS 4 FLUID OUNCES (60 TO 120 DOSES)

The herbs in this remedy pack a punch when it comes to improving fatigue significantly in people with chronic fatigue syndrome. They also offer magnesium, a mineral that is depleted in people dealing with CFS.

INGREDIENTS*

2 teaspoons nettles leaf

2 teaspoons oregano leaf

2 teaspoons parsley leaf

2 teaspoons thyme leaf

1 teaspoon alfalfa leaf

½ teaspoon red clover blossom

½ cup 80-proof vodka

Ingredients are dried unless otherwise indicated.

INSTRUCTIONS

1. In an 8-ounce glass mason jar, combine all the herbs. Pour in the vodka, seal the jar with a tight-fitting lid, and shake gently. Place the jar in a cool, dark, dry place for 4 to 6 weeks, shaking it every 1 to 2 days.

2. Strain the tincture through a fine-mesh strainer set over a bowl and use a funnel to transfer it into one amber glass dropper bottle and amber glass tincture bottles with twist caps. Label and date the bottles.

SUGGESTED USE/DOSAGE

Take 1 to 2 dropperfuls (1 to 2 mL) 2 to 3 times a day, or add to 1 cup cold or room-temperature water, for 12 weeks. Let your body rest and assess how you feel.

WARNING *Avoid nettles leaf if you are pregnant, nursing, or taking blood pressure medication.*

Rooting for You Tea

YIELDS ¾ CUP HERB MIX (FOR 24 CUPS OF TEA)

This tea is crafted from powerhouse herbal allies known for their abilities to combat inflammation, decrease fatigue, increase stamina, and support the adrenal system.

INGREDIENTS*

¼ **cup astragalus root**

3 tablespoons nettles leaf

2 tablespoons licorice root

2 tablespoons peppermint leaf

1 tablespoon ginger root

1 to 2 tablespoons honey (preferably local)

Ingredients are dried unless otherwise indicated.

INSTRUCTIONS

1. In a 16-ounce glass mason jar, combine all the herbs and seal the jar with a tight-fitting lid. Label and date the jar.

2. To prepare the tea, in a saucepan over medium heat, combine 2 tablespoons herb mix and 2 cups water. Cover the pan and heat for 20 minutes.

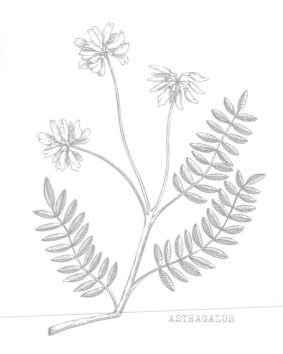

ASTRAGALUS

3. Remove from the heat and let steep for 10 minutes.

4. Strain off the herbs and pour the tea into another 16-ounce glass mason jar. Stir in the honey.

SUGGESTED USE/DOSAGE

Drink 1 to 2 cups a day or as needed.

WARNING *Avoid nettles leaf if you are pregnant, nursing, or taking blood pressure medication. Ginger should not be taken by people who have a bleeding disorder or are taking blood thinners. Do not give to children under 5 years of age.*

FIBROMYALGIA

Fibromyalgia is a disorder that causes chronic pain and tenderness throughout the body. It varies in degree of pain, but many people who live with fibromyalgia have sleep disruptions and fatigue associated with the constant state of discomfort. Many also have mental and emotional distress, memory disorder, and mood swings caused by their persistent pain. It is believed that those who are dealing with fibromyalgia have a higher awareness and perception of pain, which is compounded by the constant pain flares they experience. Herbal remedies along with other therapies can help manage fibromyalgia pain.

White Willow Tincture

YIELDS 4 FLUID OUNCES (120 DOSES)

The goal when working with fibromyalgia is taking the pain registry down. This tincture is crafted with herbs that ease pain and discomfort, contain anti-inflammatory properties, and can help prevent persistent signaling of pain in the body.

INGREDIENTS*

2 teaspoons turmeric root

1 teaspoon white willow bark

1 teaspoon astragalus root

1 teaspoon cramp bark

½ teaspoon black peppercorns (omit if you are allergic)

½ cup 80-proof vodka

Ingredients are dried unless otherwise indicated.

INSTRUCTIONS

1. In an 8-ounce glass mason jar, combine all the herbs. Pour in the vodka, seal the jar with a tight-fitting lid, and shake gently. Place the jar in a cool, dark, dry place for 6 to 8 weeks, shaking it every 1 to 2 days.

2. Strain the tincture through a fine-mesh strainer set over a bowl and use a funnel to transfer it into one amber glass dropper bottle and amber glass tincture bottles with twist caps. Label and date the bottles.

SUGGESTED USE/DOSAGE

Take 1 dropperful (1 mL) 3 times a day as needed.

WARNING *Do not take if you are pregnant, nursing, take blood thinners, or are allergic to aspirin. Do not take turmeric if you have liver or bile duct disorders. Do not give to children under 12 years of age.*

Adaptogenic "Coffee" Blend

YIELDS 1¾ CUPS PLUS 2 TABLESPOONS HERB MIX (FOR 30 CUPS OF "COFFEE")

Adaptogens help the body reduce inflammation and pain while supporting the regulation of hormones. This can help ease the stress, restless sleep, and mood swings associated with fibromyalgia. When the body is in stress mode and fibromyalgia pain is flaring, adaptogens can help the body find balance and lessen the impact of the flare.

INGREDIENTS*

½ **cup ashwagandha root**

½ **cup chicory root**

½ **cup dandelion root**

2 **tablespoons rhodiola root**

2 **tablespoons raw cacao nibs**

2 **tablespoons cinnamon chips**

Honey or other natural sweetener, for serving (optional)

Dairy or nondairy beverage, for serving (optional)

Ingredients are dried unless otherwise indicated.

INSTRUCTIONS

1. Preheat the oven to 250°F. Line a baking sheet with parchment paper.

2. Combine all the herbs on the prepared baking sheet. Bake for 2 hours, or until the cacao smells rich and chocolatey and the herbs are a nutty brown color. Let cool.

3. Grind the cooled herbs until they are the texture of ground coffee. Put the herb mix into a 16-ounce glass mason jar and seal the jar with a tight-fitting lid. Label and date the jar.

4. To prepare the "coffee," put 1 tablespoon herb mix into a tea strainer or loose-leaf tea bag and into a mug. Pour 1 cup just-boiled water over the herbs. Let steep for 5 to 10 minutes. Sweeten as desired and add dairy or nondairy as you like.

SUGGESTED USE/DOSAGE

Enjoy the same way you would enjoy your daily cup of coffee.

WARNING *Chicory should be avoided by people with irritable bowel syndrome and by pregnant and nursing people. Limit cinnamon use during pregnancy. If you take medication for diabetes, know that chicory has blood sugar–lowering properties that, if taken alongside diabetes medication, can cause blood sugar to drop dangerously low. Chicory stimulates the gallbladder and can aggravate gallstones. Be mindful if you are allergic to plants in the Asteraceae and/or Compositae families as it could trigger an allergic reaction.*

THYROID IMBALANCES (HYPER AND HYPO)

Your thyroid is a small, butterfly-shaped organ that sits at the base of your neck. It creates the hormones that help your body process fats and carbohydrates. It also regulates your weight, your energy levels, how your hair and nails grow, the health of your skin, and your internal temperature. Small but mighty is an understatement! When people have thyroid disease, their thyroid dysregulates, making too much (hyperthyroidism) or too little (hypothyroidism) of the hormones needed to support these systems in your body. Herbal support of the thyroid can help regulate hormone production and ease the symptoms and side effects of thyroid disease.

There are many herbs and plant allies that can trigger negative and harmful reactions in a person with hyperthyroidism. As with any major health condition, please check with your healthcare provider before adding any herbal or OTC remedy to your wellness practice. Your health and safety is important.

Wonderful Weeds Tincture

YIELDS 4 FLUID OUNCES (40 TO 120 DOSES)

This tincture is one of my favorites for many reasons, one being that it is made entirely out of "weeds." Cleavers, dandelions, and nettles are abundant, hardy, and easy to forage. If you have access to them in a clean foraging location, take what you need. (Use a local plant guide or plant identification app to be sure you're harvesting the correct plants.) These plants help support your thyroid health in general and can be used whether you have hyper or hypo thyroid issues.

INGREDIENTS*

¼ **cup cleavers stem and leaf**
2 **tablespoons dandelion root and leaf**
2 **tablespoons nettles leaf**
½ **cup 80-proof vodka**

Ingredients are dried unless otherwise indicated.

INSTRUCTIONS

1. In an 8-ounce glass mason jar, combine all the herbs. Pour in the vodka, seal the jar with a tight-fitting lid, and shake gently. Place the jar in a cool, dark, dry place for 4 to 6 weeks, shaking it every 1 to 3 days.

2. Strain the tincture through a fine-mesh strainer set over a bowl and use a funnel to transfer it into one

amber glass dropper bottle and amber glass tincture bottles with twist caps. Label and date the bottles.

SUGGESTED USE/DOSAGE

Take 1 to 3 dropperfuls (1 to 3 mL) 1 to 3 times a day, or add to 1 cup cold or room-temperature water. Adjust the dose as needed and discontinue use if you note any concerning side effects.

WARNING *Avoid nettles leaf if you are pregnant, nursing, or taking blood pressure medication.*

Hyperthyroid Tea

YIELDS 3 TABLESPOONS HERB MIX (FOR 9 CUPS OF TEA)

This remedy is made from herbs that help lower high thyroid hormones and help regulate thyroid function while reducing thyroid inflammation. This tea is crafted to assist in restoring healthy balance for people with hyperthyroidism.

INGREDIENTS*

1 tablespoon bugleweed flower and leaf
1 tablespoon chamomile flower
1 tablespoon nettles leaf

*Ingredients are dried unless otherwise indicated.

INSTRUCTIONS

1. In an 8-ounce glass mason jar, combine the herbs. Seal the jar with a tight-fitting lid and shake until the herbs are mixed thoroughly. Label and date the jar.

2. To prepare the tea, place 1 teaspoon herb mix into a tea strainer or loose-leaf tea bag and into a mug (or place the mix directly in the mug). Pour in 1 cup boiling water and let steep for 15 minutes. Strain as needed and sweeten if desired.

SUGGESTED USE/DOSAGE

Drink 1 cup once or twice a day as needed, paying close attention to how your body responds to the remedy and adjust the dose as needed. Discontinue use if you notice any concerning side effects.

WARNING *Avoid nettles leaf if you are pregnant, nursing, or taking blood pressure medication. Be mindful if you are allergic to plants in the Asteraceae and/or Compositae families as chamomile could trigger an allergic reaction.*

Iodine-Rich Kombu Furikake

YIELDS HEAPING ¾ CUP (12 DOSES)

Key markers of hypothyroidism include a lack of iodine and selenium. This herbal remedy is rich in iodine from sea vegetables as well as selenium from sesame seeds and mushroom powder. Black cumin seeds have been shown to positively affect the levels of the thyroid hormones thyroxine (T4) and triiodothyronine (T3) in people with hypothyroidism. Not bad for a yummy snack!

INGREDIENTS

2 tablespoons black sesame seeds

1 tablespoon white sesame seeds

2 teaspoons black cumin seeds

½ cup kombu flakes

1 tablespoon shiitake mushroom powder

½ teaspoon coarse sea salt or Himalayan rock salt

INSTRUCTIONS

1. Preheat the oven to 350°F. Line a baking sheet with parchment paper.

2. Spread the black sesame seeds, white sesame seeds, and black cumin seeds on the prepared baking sheet in a single layer. Roast until the seeds are lightly toasted and begin to smell nutty, 8 to 10 minutes, stirring every few minutes. Let cool completely so they don't wilt the kombu.

3. In the small bowl, stir together the cooled seeds, kombu flakes, mushroom powder, and salt. Transfer to an 8-ounce glass mason jar and seal the jar with a tight-fitting lid. Label and date the jar. Store with your other spices.

SUGGESTED USE/DOSAGE

Furikake is a delicious seasoning that comes from Japanese culture. Use 1 tablespoon per serving on popcorn, rice bowls, sushi, fish, noodles or, if you're anything like me, right out of the palm of your hand. Be well!

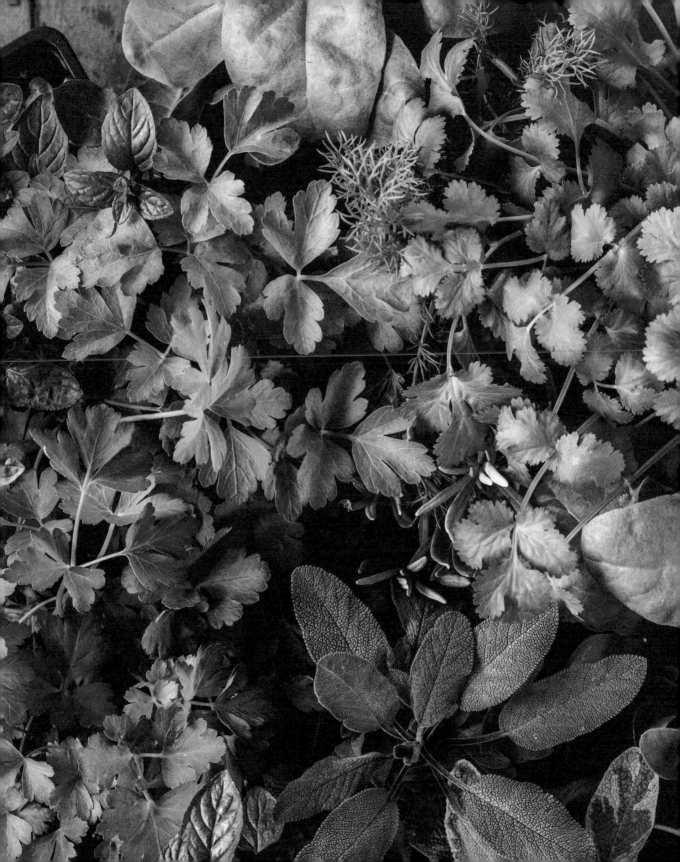

Resources

I wish I could list every one of my favorite books and herbal supplies sources for you, but that could be an entire other book! Here are a few of my favorites:

Books

Botanical Safety Handbook (second edition) by Zoë Garnder and Michael McGuffin (eds)

Herbal Contraindications and Drug Interactions: Plus Herbal Adjuncts with Medicines (fourth edition) by Francis Brinker

Alchemy of Herbs: Transform Everyday Ingredients into Foods and Remedies That Heal by Rosalee De La Foret

The Modern Herbal Dispensatory: A Medicine-Making Guide by Thomas Easley and Steven H. Horne

Herbs for Children's Health: How to Make and Use Gentle Herbal Remedies for Soothing Common Ailments by Rosemary Gladstar

Herbs for Common Ailments: How to Make and Use Herbal Remedies for Home Health Care by Rosemary Gladstar

Rosemary Gladstar's Family Herbal: A Guide to Living Life with Energy, Health, and Vitality by Rosemary Gladstar

Rosemary Gladstar's Medicinal Herbs: A Beginner's Guide by Rosemary Gladstar

Medical Herbalism: The Science Principles and Practices of Herbal Medicine by David Hoffman

Handbook of African Medicinal Plants by Maurice M. Iwu

Working the Roots: Over 400 Years of Traditional African American Healing by Michele Lee

Hormone Intelligence: The Complete Guide to Calming Hormone Chaos and Restoring Your Body's Natural Blueprint for Well-Being by Aviva Romm

IWÍGARA: The Kinship of Plants and People by Enrique Salmón

Herb, Nutrient, and Drug Interactions: Clinical Implications and Therapeutic Strategies by Mitchell Bebel Stargrove, Jonathan Treasure, and Dwight L. McKee

African American Herbalism: A Practical Guide to Healing Plants and Folk Traditions by Lucretia VanDyke

Taking Charge of Your Fertility: The Definitive Guide to Natural Birth Control, Pregnancy Achievement, and Reproductive Health (updated edition) by Toni Weschler

Organizations

Herb Rally
www.herbrally.com

Herb Rally is an online hub for the herbal community. It helps connect herbalists across the country and updates the community with news about events, podcasts, courses, and more.

Mountain Rose Herbs
www.mountainroseherbs.com

Mountain Rose Herbs is not merely a supplier of herbs and herbal medicine crafting materials—it is an amazing resource for herbalists in all stages of their practice. Founded by acclaimed author and herbalist Rosemary Gladstar in 1987, Mountain Rose Herbs has worked to be at the forefront of sustainable, ethical, and ecologically responsible herbal business practices. They have multiple certifications—from organic and non-GMO to safe foraging and zero waste. The company has also started the Free Herbalism Project and the Seed Stewardship Project, giving away packets of endangered seeds free to raise awareness about endangered plants and ways to protect them.

North American Native Plant Society
www.nanps.org

Founded in Toronto, Canada, NANPS is committed to studying, conserving, and cultivating native plant habitats in wild areas of North America and restoring indigenous flora to developed areas.

The Herbal Academy
www.theherbalacademy.com

The Herbal Academy is an online educational space as well as an amazing resource for herbalists in all stages of their journey. Their goal is to guide people toward affordable and accessible herbal skills, offering training for everyone from the novice at-home crafter to the person seeking to create herbal medicine professionally.

United Plant Savers
www.unitedplantsavers.org

A prominent voice for protecting our herbal allies, United Plant Savers teaches people about at-risk plants and low-impact harvesting practices. It also maintains a global network of conservation lands and botanical sanctuaries to preserve biodiversity and plant knowledge of important at-risk medicinal plants and plants that are important for food, craft, and sacred ceremony.

References

De La Foret, Rosalee. 2017. *Alchemy of Herbs: Transform Everyday Ingredients into Foods and Remedies That Heal.* Carlsbad, CA: Hay House.

Easley, Thomas, and Horne, Steven H. 2016. *The Modern Herbal Dispensatory: A Medicine-Making Guide.* Berkeley, CA: North Atlantic Books.

Gladstar, Rosemary. 2014. *Herbs for Common Ailments: How to Make and Use Herbal Remedies for Home Health Care.* North Adams, MA: Storey Publishing, LLC.

Gladstar, Rosemary. 2001. *Rosemary Gladstar's Family Herbal: A Guide to Living Life with Energy, Health, and Vitality.* North Adams, MA: Storey Publishing, LLC.

Gladstar, Rosemary. 2012. *Rosemary Gladstar's Medicinal Herbs: A Beginner's Guide.* North Adams, MA: Storey Publishing, LLC.

Hoffman, David. 2003. *Medical Herbalism: The Science Principles and Practices of Herbal Medicine.* Rochester, VT: Healing Arts Press.

Iwu, Maurice M. 2014. *Handbook of African Medicinal Plants.* Boca Raton, FL: CRC Press.

Lee, Michele. 2017. *Working the Roots: Over 400 Years of Traditional African American Healing.* Oakland, CA: Wadastick Publishers.

New York University. October 14, 2021. "Americans Are Eating More Ultra-Processed Foods." www.nyu.edu/about/news-publications/news/2021/october/ultra-processed-foods.html.

Romm, Aviva. 2021. *Hormone Intelligence: The Complete Guide to Calming Hormone Chaos and Restoring Your Body's Natural Blueprint for Well-Being.* San Francisco: HarperOne.

Salmón, Enrique. 2020. *IWÍGARA: The Kinship of Plants and People.* Portland, OR: Timber Press.

VanDyke, Lucretia. 2023. *African American Herbalism: A Practical Guide to Healing Plants and Folk Traditions.* New York: Ulysses Press.

Weschler, Toni. 2015. *Taking Charge of Your Fertility: The Definitive Guide to Natural Birth Control, Pregnancy Achievement, and Reproductive Health, Updated Ed.* New York: William Morrow Paperbacks.

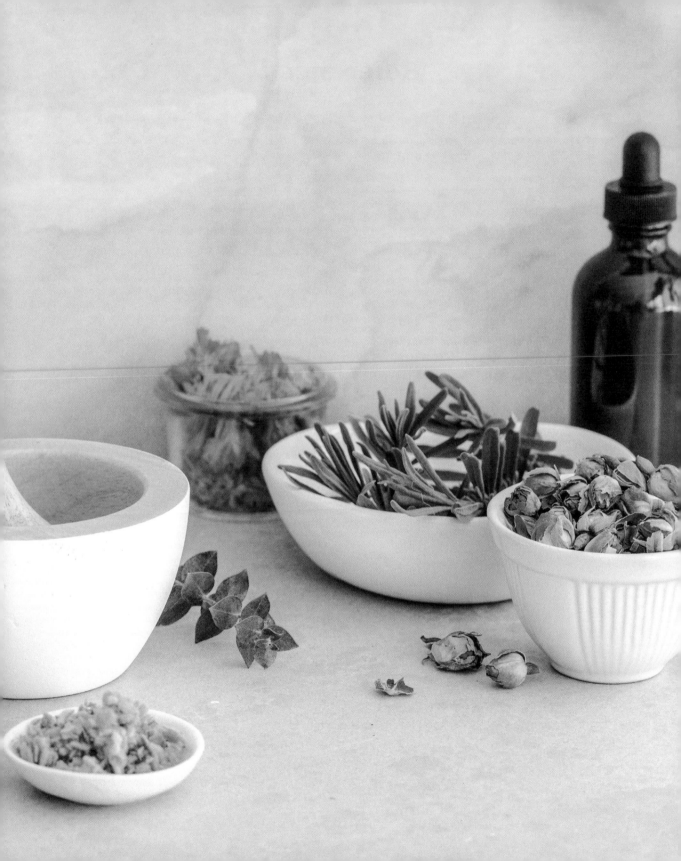

Index

Acknowledgments

As an herbal practitioner, there are so many people whose conversation and knowledge have allowed me to grow in my skills. I am grateful for these interactions, even if I cannot name everyone. I want to acknowledge my mom, who has shared the wisdom of her mother and her matrilineal folk medicine knowledge with me through our African and Indigenous blood-lines/heritage. It is what started my journey into honing the art of plant healing. I will forever be grateful to my ancestors for the knowledge they carried and for what I have been able to gather from the parts I was given. And I want to thank my children who listen to me prattle on about plant medicine and who actually use the skills I have shared with them. I know that they will continue to carry this Sacred practice into the future.

About the Author

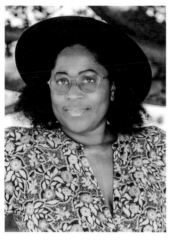

Ruth A. Blanding is a modern herbalist, wellness practitioner, and birth worker who lives and works with her heart and passions strongly rooted in her multicultural ancestry. She enjoys mindfully combining the time-trusted "grandmother wisdom" learned from the Earth and nature practices of her African and Native American ancestries with her love for solid, factual, whole-being centered care. Often, she feels as though she is an Intuitive and a Conduit of Communication and Knowledge with the Universe, the Elders, and the Ancestors. She frequently finds herself helping others find and live as their most authentic and highest selves and in their highest purpose.

Ruth holds close to deep traditions that span back into her ancestral lineage and blends them seamlessly with her lifelong study and sixteen years of practice. She comes from a long line of healers, shamans, and medicine people and has always had a deep connection with the healing magic of herbs, the mindful touch of hands to body, and the deep meditative healing practices that sit in the body-memory of every living being.

All her years gathering skills and knowledge have led Ruth to stand in her belief that every being can heal and grow, and that each person has the capacity to be a conduit of that healing process for themselves and their loved ones. It is her goal to support, educate, inspire, and gently guide all those with whom she works.

When not working, Ruth can be found writing, herb crafting, playing in the dirt, and enjoying a simple and beautiful life with the four of her six children who still live at home.

Hi there,

We hope you enjoyed *Herbal Medicine for Modern Life*. If you have any questions or concerns about your book, or have received a damaged copy, please contact customerservice@penguinrandomhouse.com. We're here and happy to help.

Also, please consider writing a review on your favorite retailer's website to let others know what you thought of the book!

Sincerely,
The Zeitgeist Team